What healthcare professionals and reviewers are saying about *Emergency Room Survival Guide:*

"BoomER Emergency Room Survival Guide for Baby Boomers and Older Folks is a primer that should be on the bookshelves of not just baby boomers or older adults, but any family member or caregiver. It provides essential, specific information from physicians who document common emergency room issues and how patients can be proactive in handling sudden emergencies and critical care treatment.... BoomER is very highly recommended as an essential consumer guide that nobody should be without."

Midwest Book Review, Diane Donovan, Senior Book Reviewer

"BoomER Emergency Room Survival Guide should be mandatory reading for all who are in the business of caring for the elderly, whether a professional in a medical setting or caring for a mother or father at home. Readers will pick up pearls of info they can use in real life."

Robert Ziomek, BSN, MSN, Owner and Manager, Lovin Manor Assisted Living Homes Scottsdale, AZ

"I wholeheartedly recommend this book to every adult, no matter their age or health condition. Do yourself a favor and get a copy. Read the book and then take action that stands to render better care for you when you find yourself as an ER patient. This book is a gift to the general public and to health care providers. I am recommending it to all my family, friends and colleagues."

Paige Hector, LMSW, Clinical Educator & Consultant, Paige Ahead Healthcare Education & Consulting, L.L.C.

"BoomER Emergency Room Survival Guide is an extraordinary and compelling insider's account of the risks we all face in the event of common medical crises. Nobody is immune from suffering a potentially unforeseen and life-threatening event. Therefore, this book could be regarded as a wake up call for a vast audience that includes aging adults,those who love them, caregivers, and all healthcare workers who care for older adults."

Maribeth Gallagher, DNP, FAAN, Dementia Program Director, Hospice of the Valley

BoomER

EMERGENCY ROOM
SURVIVAL
GUIDE
FOR BABY BOOMERS
AND OLDER FOLKS

BoomER

EMERGENCY ROOM
SURVIVAL
GUIDE
FOR BABY BOOMERS
AND OLDER FOLKS

ROBERT DERLET, MD
& JOEL COHEN, MD

ENDLESS KNOT PRESS
Scottsdale, Arizona

ISBN Print Edition: 978-0-9963090-0-4
Library of Congress Control Number: 2015917576

Published by Endless Knot Press, LLC
Mailing Address: PO Box 7904
Cave Creek, AZ 85327

Publisher Website: www.endlessknotpress.com
Book Website: **www.emergencyroomsurvivalbookforolderadults.com**

Cover graphic design by Damonza
Cover photo by FlutterDshutter
Edited by Joel Cohen, MD

Bulk Sales:
NOTE: Geriatric organizations, hospices, home health agencies, assisted living and skilled nursing facilities or organizations, and healthcare-related student education organizations:
Discounts are available to purchase this book in larger quantities to distribute to employees or students as an educational tool, and to offer as a gift of organization membership or event attendance.
For information about bulk sales please contact Endless Knot Press by email at endlessknotpress@gmail.com or call 480-818-7845. Also check our website: www.endlessknotpress.com.

PUBLISHER'S NOTE AND DISCLAIMER

Any medical guidance in this book should be used for informational and educational purposes only. Information contained in this book and on the book website (emergencyroomsurvivalbookforolderadults.com) serves only as supplement to, not substitute for, a professional medical evaluation including physical examination, medical history, necessary diagnostic tests, and discussion about the best treatment approach for each individual. Readers must also use their own best judgment during bouts of acute illness. Book content should not be misconstrued as medical diagnosis or personal physician treatment advice. Remember to ask your treating doctors wise questions. Elicit clear, thorough and understandable explanations for any recommended tests or treatments.

Names or identifying details of individuals mentioned in this book may have been changed to protect their privacy.

Contents

INTRODUCTION
NOSOCOMEPHOBIA CURED BY PATIENT-POWER?

HEALTHCARE SYSTEMS ACROSS the globe are in trouble — from emergency rooms to hospitals to primary care. Just a few key concerns: Older, sicker populations; inundated emergency rooms; deadly and invisible hospital dangers; astronomical costs; technology worship; compassion and quality-of-life considerations have become extinct dinosaurs amidst complex medical care for aging adults.

This book informs readers about hidden dangers in emergency rooms and hospitals, offering practical tips and solutions. Solutions— *that* is what BoomER is about. Emergency rooms and hospitals do save countless lives and provide exemplary care much of the time. That is, when patients use the emergency room or hospital wisely, and when physicians and nurses make sensible medical decisions in the best interest of patients. Even under ideal conditions, hazards abound in those sterile, white corridors. Some risks are avoidable, while other perils strike hard and fast like a speeding train without headlights or horn. Treatment risk is ever-present and inevitable. Unexpected and undesirable outcomes befall patients when tests are ordered, procedures are performed and medications are prescribed – all during a chaotic emergency room visit or hospitalization.

Emergency room and hospital care can be improved if people learn the weaknesses in the system and adopt a proactive approach. Never utter the words, "Whatever you say, doc." The mission and goal of BoomER is simple: "Patient-Power." Readers will find this book chock full of valuable tools and advice to help people get quality care during medical crises. This book might help to reduce chances for calamities in care. Caregivers and healthcare workers who care for frail elderly and disabled folks will also find BoomER an indispensible resource.

Before embarking on our journey to improve future care for older adults, let us take a quick look back at the recent past. In 1976, a Los Angeles County doctors' strike propagated waves of panic and fear across that desert city. Would many people die as healers played hooky and stayed home? Perhaps illness would creep like a plague, infecting thousands of Los Angeles residents and striking down its victims without mercy? As things turned out, the death rate *dropped* by 18 percent during that doctors' strike!

That same year, doctors went on strike for 52 days in Bogota, Columbia. Did medical panic and pandemonium prevail? No, the death rate *dropped* by 35 percent! In Israel, circa 1983, doctors went on strike for more than 3 months but the death rate did not increase during that period of uncertainty.

Physicians and other healthcare providers do wonderful work every day, particularly in emergency departments across the globe. Medical treatments, drugs, surgery, technology, hospitals and procedures are, however, a two-edged scalpel. Medical care can cure, but can also cut, maim and lacerate. Procedures and tests that patients undergo and the pills people pop pose dangers, risks and side effects that must be weighed against potential benefits.

Interestingly, it has been reported that Dr Richard Smith, former editor of the British Medical Journal, stated that visiting a hospital can be more dangerous than bungee jumping!

Those doctors' strikes from decades past send us a clear message today – hospitals, emergency rooms and doctors collectively provide the best of care… and the *worst* of care. Not unlike the barbaric bloodletting and skull trephining treatments of centuries past, drug treatments and invasive procedures take their toll on patients. In fact, a new study published in the *Journal of Public Safety* estimated that as many as 440,000 people in the United States die from medical errors, bad reactions or complications every year! That is four times the estimate by the Institute of Medicine's 1999 report titled, *To Err is Human*. This previous patient safety and risk report created quite a clamor over a decade ago!

Ultimately, it is each person's responsibility to ensure he or she is informed and receives patient-centered care that suits individual needs and preferences. Good medical care means striking a balance of risks versus rewards versus personal preferences for care. It is true a hospital and doctor can be your best allies when you suffer from serious illness. Yet, there is also undeniable truth to the adage, "The hospital is the worst place to be when you are sick." This is particularly accurate for frail and chronically ill older adults since this group is most susceptible to hospital hazards. Older bodies simply have less capacity to withstand bodily stress and insult.

One clear lesson you should learn from this book: It is *not* always better to get tests and accept treatments and to undergo surgical procedures. Every treatment and test has its pitfalls, complications, mess-ups, unexpected consequences and risks.

Consider life expectancy relative to technology. The United States is king when it comes to use of technology. So why was the United States ranked only 26th in life expectancy worldwide, according to a 2013 Organisation for Economic Co-operation and Development report? Austria boasts a two-year longer life expectancy, for example, yet performs half the MRI exams as the United States. There is clearly a disconnect between overzealous use of technology and procedures and actual benefit to patients. In truth, these glorious medical gizmos are not magic wands. They pose significant hazards to patients.

Considering all the tests, treatments and other dangers that await patients in emergency rooms and hospitals worldwide, it is no wonder many people have a fear of going to the hospital or emergency room. The elderly arguably suffer from the greatest fear of hospitals, worried they will die there or never return to their home and current quality of lifestyle. Believe it or not, there is a word for this fear – nosocomephobia, the extreme fear of hospitals. It has been reported that former president Richard Nixon may have had nosecomephobia, having been quoted as saying, "If I go to a hospital, I'm fairly sure I won't come out of it alive." Fear of modern-day hospitals, however, is *not* unrealistic or unreasonable. Emergency rooms, the major gateways into hospitals, are also fraught with real and ever-present dangers.

It may surprise you to know that each and every patient has the *most* power to minimize treatment risks. Believe it! A 2015 physician survey published in *Academic Emergency Medicine* found that 97 percent of emergency room doctors order unnecessary tests out of fear of getting sued for a missed diagnosis. What's more, many university and teaching hospitals subject ER patients to needless tests and procedures based upon automatic algorithms of care that must be done all the time, without regard to patient safety, comfort or preference. For instance, a victim of a car accident will likely be wheeled in by ambulance with standard-protocol hard body-board and neck-collar in place. That car accident victim, at some hospitals, will likely be subjected to multiple x-rays or CT scans, and possibly a bladder catheter, intravenous lines and other invasive and uncomfortable procedures – even if that person apparently sustained less than serious injuries! Why do all this? It is hospital protocol to avoid 'mistakes' in care as well as liability. Doctors remain at the mercy of their own malpractice fears and imposed hospital protocols. Sometimes it is financial gain that motivates or obligates doctors and hospitals to overuse tests and procedures. Only the patient has the power to quash the epidemic of risky and avoidable tests and treatments.

You might ask: "How can I, a sick patient at the mercy of a behemoth hospital, be empowered to avoid unnecessary and questionable tests or treatments?" Use your "Patient-Power." Just say "No!" to iffy tests and treatments. Ask the right questions and your doctor's approach and tune might change regarding ordering that procedure, test or medication. You will be equipped with "Patient-Power" tools throughout the pages of BoomER. Did you know these patient powers are expressly stated in the universal Patient Bill of Rights?

To refuse medical treatment even if it is recommended by their physician(s); and to be informed about their medical condition, the risks and benefits of treatment and appropriate alternatives.

Read on to learn about "Informed Consent Question-Kits" (**IC Q-Kits**) containing key questions that can empower patients. Also in the pages that follow:

- A new educational approach to help folks recall and identify stroke symptoms, and to identify personal risk factors
- A novel, descriptive way to more accurately recognize if you may be suffering from a serious heart condition

- Taking the dread out of someday being dead: Advance directives explained the "Die Happy" way. It may shock you to know most people, including many healthcare providers, misunderstand Do Not Resuscitate forms and the end-of-life care process.
- Help for caregivers in early identification of red-flag signs of serious illness. This vital resource can help frail elders avoid some hospitalizations.

Planning Ahead: Seeking Care in a Drowning System

The first step in getting excellent emergency care is advance planning. You hang smoke detectors and map out a fire drill to plan for fire ravaging your home. You even write out a Last Will and Testament in case the unthinkable happens. But have you thought about which hospital emergency room to go to for a heart attack or stroke? Chances for sudden illness are greater than for a house fire, yet most people do little to plan for medical calamity. You develop crushing chest pain, for example. Which hospital emergency room has the best capabilities to save your life and which hospital ER might be less effective in treating your massive heart attack?

Do your research based upon guidance offered in this book and using procedure and hospital ranking websites. Develop a solid plan of action *now*. You do not want to make key healthcare decisions in a cloud of panic during a crisis. Where did I put our family doctor's on-call phone number? Which hospital should I drive to for severe food poisoning? For a heart attack? What is the quickest route there? Should I call for an ambulance? "I couldn't be having a stroke"—what are the signs and symptoms? Does the hospital know I want only comfort measures for grandma who is at the end of her life? How can I arrange for that wish to be honored?

Let's face it, sooner or later you or a loved one will end up prone and vulnerable on a hard stretcher. How bad can emergency care actually be? Must I really plan far in advance? In Truth, emergency rooms have become chaotic and unpredictable. Doctors and nurses are overwhelmed and overworked because of overcrowding. Medical care and technology have grown complex and risky – and overused!. This dangerous brew breeds errors and oversights, side effects and complications. Minimize your risk of becoming a medical statistic.

If you need further convincing, the highly regarded American College of Emergency Physicians has released its 2014 Report Card on emergency care in the United States. The national grade was a barely passing D+!

Put together your own plan for medical calamity today. Start by entering your key information on the interior front or back cover of this printed book for quick reference (if available in your edition). Refer to Appendix A in the back of the book for the nuts and bolts of planning ahead for medical emergencies. Read on for a treasure trove of guidance pearls.

Learn how to be proactive and feel the "Patient-Power." Then research the pros and cons of your local hospitals, emergency departments and urgent care facilities. University teaching hospitals are more likely to offer the latest technology, procedures and complex surgeries, especially after hours and overnight; however these treatments can be overused when always available. Reputable community hospitals offer excellent customer service for routine procedures or basic emergencies like appendicitis, dehydration or less serious injuries. The downside in a community hospital is that many specialists, tests and procedures are less available during night hours and weekends.

Research if your hospital ranks high in successful heart procedures or fewer infections. Does the emergency room offer a special stroke treatment center or geriatric care unit? Speak to friends and leaders in your community about their experiences with local care facilities such as hospitals, urgent care centers, primary care providers and specialists. Even ask others for recommendations about local pharmacies that offer better customer service, education and pricing for medications. Perhaps most importantly, develop a good relationship with a trusted primary care doctor or appropriate specialist who can see you quickly when needed and give you crucial guidance during a medical crisis. Use the information in this book, combined with your doctor's guidance, to allay your fears. Those common fears include that of going to emergency rooms ("ER-angst") and hospital paranoia ("hospanoia") as I have labeled these worries. Read on and feel your fears gradually melt away as you absorb a mega-dose of patient empowerment.

SECTION II

WHY ALL THE FUSS ABOUT CARE OF OLDER ADULTS IN EMERGENCY ROOMS? THE GERIATRIC DELUGE

THE DELUGE HAS already begun. Older adults account for nearly 25 million annual emergency department visits in the United States and up to 20 percent of Canadian emergency department visits. The "Geriatric Deluge" or "Geri-D" as I call it, will achieve nothing less than tsunami status in the coming three decades as the global elderly population is predicted to hit between one and 1.5 billion folks over age 60.

Why all the fuss? The elderly present many challenges in the emergency care setting. Older folks frequently try to avoid the emergency room and hospital because they fear dying there or never returning home. The tradeoff is that older folks are generally sicker, oftentimes seriously ill, when they do get to an emergency room. Seniors are more likely to arrive by ambulance and get admitted into the hospital. They spend more time in the ER while being subjected to increasingly complex testing, and are more likely to need a hard-to-get intensive care unit bed. For the silver-haired crowd, it is not lack of an available primary care doctor that leads to emergency room visits. The primary care or nursing home doctor, in fact, commonly *sends* older patients to the emergency department – even before performing an evaluation.

It is counterintuitive that older folks frequently get *worse* after arrival at the emergency room. A 2013 international study published in the *Annals of Emergency Medicine* looked at the functional and cognitive abilities of elderly ER patients over 74 years of age before the visit and after arrival in an emergency room. Seven countries were represented including emergency rooms in Australia, Belgium, Canada, Germany, Iceland, India and Sweden. Before the visit, 46 percent of seniors had some functional dependency. After arrival in the emergency room, 67 percent needed assistance with some daily living activities. Those who needed help with walking nearly doubled from before the ER visit to after arrival. Furthermore, a recent Canadian study found that nearly one in 10 emergency room patients over age 85 remained mired in ER chaos longer than twenty-four hours, placing these frail, elderly folks at great risk for medication errors and other adverse events.

Difficult to Diagnose

Studies have also found that older adults are less likely to get an accurate diagnosis in the emergency room. A few reasons: less typical signs of disease in seniors, other complicating chronic illnesses, and too many medications. In fact, up to 20 percent of older folks who wind up in an emergency room have vague complaints such as "weakness" or "not feeling well." This further challenges an ER doctor's ability to get a correct diagnosis.

In addition to multiple chronic illnesses, less typical disease presentations, and a pharmacopeia of medications, additional challenges exist that may hinder chances for older adults to receive quality emergency care: weakened kidney function leading to greater risk for drug toxicity, and communication difficulty due to memory loss, confusion or hearing and vision impairment. These obstacles can lead to delayed care, treatment complications or outright misdiagnosis.

Seniors who are frail and arrive from nursing homes or assisted living settings can cause still greater diagnostic difficulty for emergency room doctors. These elderly patients have complex medical histories and are time-consuming to care for. Their complex medical histories may not be known to the ER doctor and records and pertinent history are often unavailable. What is more, many emergency room doctors and nurses lack special training in caring for seniors.

Risk factors have been identified that portend poor outcomes from an emergency room visit. They include older age, recent hospitalization or

ER visit, impaired functional ability with daily activities, living alone and social isolation. A senior's dependence on others for daily activities may be the most important risk factor for poor outcomes after an emergency room visit.

The Perfect Emergency Room Visit

What if we could build a dam, tighten a spigot, and slow the geriatric patient rapids to a lazy-river-like pace. What, then, would the perfect emergency room experience be like for older adults? The United States now boasts over fifty emergency departments nationwide that specialize in treating *only* older adults. I call them *SilvERs*. A few of the accoutrements that a silver-haired guest might encounter at a SilvER include thicker stretcher mattresses to reduce discomfort and pressure ulcers; gentle sun-simulating lighting by day and softer, non-glare lighting by night; some degree of peace and quiet; orienting large clocks and calming wall paintings; floors less likely to cause slips and falls; and geriatric-trained healthcare workers. Sadly, less than one percent of medical students go on to specialize in geriatrics because older folks tend to be a sick population, require high paperwork demands, and offer few financial incentives for doctors to care for time-sapping sick elders.

But the ideal emergency room visit is also one in which an older adult suffers from serious, *acute* illness and whose personal choice is for hospital care. This older adult will be aware that risky, invasive procedures and more aggressive treatments may be part of the emergency care process. When older folks, especially frail elderly, get admitted into a hospital, bad things can happen. So it is crucial for benefits to outweigh possible risks of a hospital visit.

Trinity Health has been a pioneer in geriatric emergency room care. Consider this quote from the Trinity Health website:

"We thought seniors would say that they were interested in a more efficient, higher-tech experience," says Bonnie Mahon, Holy Cross' senior director for medical, surgical and senior services, who led a half dozen focus groups to learn what they thought would help improve their emergency room experience. "Instead, they said, 'Keep me warm, informed, and let my family stay with me to advocate.' "

Sadly, most emergency rooms do not do focus groups to find out what type of care seniors want most.

Name-Calling Can be Harmful

Too many emergency care providers and doctors-in-training in the United States, Canada, United Kingdom, Australia and around the globe harbor negative attitudes toward elderly patients. Commonly used derogatory names for sick, older adults that had been used for decades include "GOMER (get out of my emergency room)," "bed-blocker," "acopia (cannot cope)," and others. These terms depict the elderly as hopeless cases who take up much valuable doctor time with little chance for positive outcome. Chronically-ill seniors who are sent to emergency rooms from nursing homes have taken the brunt of these attitudes. These frail folks are more likely to have vague ailments and limited ability to communicate. Some in the medical field have used derogatory terms such as "practicing veterinary medicine" when caring for frail and vulnerable older adults.

Fortunately, the dignified care of elders has become a more established part of medical care nowadays, but bias against older folks remains. Ageism can surely hamper care of the elderly if these patients are considered by some to be hopeless cases and time-wasters. First, treatable illnesses can go undiagnosed when these seniors are ignored and considered hopeless cases needing only social services. Second, with dismissive attitudes and demeaning labels, there cannot be truly compassionate care.

Older Adults at Great Risk

A multitude of risks await older folks in emergency rooms: lack of adequate geriatric training for ER staff; poor design of emergency departments that promote confusion and loss of dignity for elders; inadequate equipment to accommodate special needs such as hard stretchers that cause pain and can quickly lead to bed sores; and high risk for loss of physical function, mental alertness, and quality of life in the days and weeks *following* an ER visit. It is also concerning that many frail residents of nursing homes and assisted living are reflexively shipped out to emergency rooms before an urgent doctor or nurse practitioner evaluation is performed. Many of these less than life-threatening ailments could have been handled without hospitalization and the hazards of an emergency department visit. This is particularly true for skilled nursing home residents who are sent from a facility that should be able to offer more advanced levels of treatment.

A balance-scale approach must always be used in deciding if an emergency room visit is needed and whether any other options are available. More importantly, we must strive for early detection and treatment of simmering sickness in seniors before reaching the point of medical crisis and calamity.

SECTION III

SIX EYE-OPENING TOPICS WITH SHOCKING EMERGENCY ROOM (ER) CARE ANECDOTES

I. MAN WITH ABDOMINAL PAIN: WILL HE LIVE OR DIE?

THE BELLY PAIN felt like a sledgehammer. That was the first thought the man had when intense abdominal pain struck his healthy 50-year-old body. In a humorous way, it reminded him of the carnival sledgehammer game that tests your strength. Only this hammer seemed to swing square into the man's upper abdomen and its power would have surely rung the bell. He writhed from side to side trying to remove himself from the affliction that assaulted his muscular body. He seemed to be squirming out from his body like a snake shedding skin. The man tried to shed a layer of agony but nothing helped. Soon his torso was soaked in sweat and a spasm of nausea overtook him.

"Must be a bad ulcer," he guessed, though he never had any serious stomach ailments. No big deal, he always had a high threshold for pain so he could handle this, he thought. The ailing man canceled his workday and waited it out. Soon the sharp pain subsided into a steady, deep gnawing. In fact, he kept an evening business appointment and then played some ping pong with a friend that night. The menu for the next few days would be chicken soup— mostly the broth— and stomach acid-lowering medication off the shelf.

After a stormy few days the pain seemed to finally subside. He awoke

Monday morning ready to conquer the world and catch up on missed work. The man ate a light brunch consisting of Greek yogurt, a banana and a slice of cheese then did a light workout at the gym. He felt well.

The calm, however, did not last long. Ninety minutes after brunch, the sledgehammer struck again – harder and harder with each assault on his upper abdomen. The bell must have rung ten times. The wave of nausea returned along with an expanding ache in the back. His body squirmed and writhed like a cobra swaying to a charmer's flute.

When the pain let up and became bearable, the man drove himself to a trusted community emergency room that was part of a teaching hospital system. He had reached his limit. Seeking medical help was long overdue. The man managed to use his smartphone to search the hospital's website which posted emergency room wait times. The smaller satellite hospital reported a far shorter wait than the main hospital trauma centers. After all, it was Monday – predictably one of the busiest days of the week in any emergency department.

The ER doctor, like Sherlock Holmes in a white coat, evaluated the sick man and was perplexed: did he suffer uncommon symptoms of a heart attack? Problems in the chest can cause abdominal pain and abdominal ailments can sometimes cause perceived chest symptoms. If this was an atypical picture of a heart attack, his young heart muscle would be dying cell by cell: there was no time to lose. The doctor quickly ordered an electrocardiogram (EKG) and blood tests to check for heart muscle damage. This was crucial since clot-dissolving drugs and emergency catheter procedures can stop a heart attack in its tracks. The pain peaked. A morphine haze finally brought some reprieve as the EKG wires were attached to his chest and limbs. The ER doctor anxiously awaited the readout of squiggly lines that can reveal the secrets of hidden heart damage beneath the chest wall.

In truth, this man had no risk factors for heart disease, nor did he experience true chest pain or difficulty breathing. He felt *better* after light exercise; an oxygen-starved heart would protest with worse symptoms if stressed by exercise. There was no heart disease in his family history and his diet was quite good. There was no diabetes, high blood pressure, high cholesterol or smoking history. The doctor was not surprised when he saw a normal EKG and heart muscle enzymes.

Next on the diagnosis menu was a possible gallbladder attack. The patient's pain twice seemed to crescendo soon after eating. "Was a gallstone rumbling through his bile duct?" the doctor wondered. That would be a tidy, simple answer to this medical puzzle but as is often the case in medicine – there are rarely easy answers. Ultrasound: normal. Perhaps that sledgehammer was a kidney stone since his urine had in it a few microscopic cells of blood? Kidney stones pack enough pain-punch to qualify as a sledgehammer and sometimes cause mostly abdominal symptoms. After all, he did suffer more back pain while in the emergency room, back pain being more typical of kidney stone agony.

Result: the kidney ultrasound was normal too. The experienced emergency room doctor knew a small kidney stone or gallstone might not show up on an ultrasound. The doctor next ordered a more accurate abdominal CT scan. When the ER doctor told his enigmatic patient the scan results, it sent the man into a tailspin. The details did not compute. Panic settled over his stretcher like threatening cumulonimbus clouds.

The head of the pancreas showed vague swelling and abnormality. If it was pancreatic cancer, the dazed man realized, he had perhaps a few months to live. There would be no 25th wedding anniversary trip to Hawaii with his wife. The ER doctor reassured him that pancreatic cancer would not usually cause a sledgehammer-type symptom picture. It was small consolation. "Perhaps I'm one of the unusual cases?" His internal sense of dread was set ablaze.

The abnormalities did not end there. Next abnormal finding on CT scan: possible inflammation of the duodenum, a key part of the small intestine that wraps around the pancreas. The ER doctor now wondered if his patient had an ulcer after all. Or was that inflammation related to the pancreas problem? The medical mystery grew. Third abnormal CT scan finding: possible aneurysm or swelling of the Celiac Artery, a major artery within the abdomen centered between the pancreas and duodenum.

The sledgehammer pain had returned only it now whacked the ill man's brain. He was in shock. Healthy one day but today he may have two potentially serious ailments erupting inside his abdomen. He squeezed his wife's hand as if to say, "Fasten your seatbelt, this ER ride is going to get real bumpy." It seemed to them there would not be any happy ending to this story.

A specialist performed an endoscopy the following morning, a procedure in which the doctor looks inside the stomach and intestine with a fiber-optic scope. Within fifteen minutes they knew even less. The test was completely normal. No ulcer or intestinal inflammation. Back to the drawing board. Later that morning, however, the ill man's blood test results offered the first concrete clue: his pancreas enzymes were high. This suggested pancreatitis, a serious inflammation of the pancreas. But what would have caused this? The two most common causes of pancreatitis are either gallstones or alcohol abuse. The man rarely drank alcohol so perhaps a tiny stone remained hidden in the tiny tubular chutes connecting the gallbladder to the intestine? A specialized MRI using contrast dye could check that to exclude small stones and tumors of the gallbladder, pancreas and surrounding areas. There were mounting radiation exposure risks at this point, but because of the severity of his symptoms the man decided these tests needed to be done to get a diagnosis.

Meanwhile, the concern about an aneurysm in the man's major abdominal artery loomed large. As the prospect of pancreatic cancer seemed less likely, worry that an aneurysm could burst and he could bleed to death took center stage. A vascular surgeon was called in to consult and told the worried man it was possible the radiologist "over-read" the CT scan since the artery size was borderline enlarged. The only way to know with some certainty was to have yet another exposure to x-ray radiation with a CT scan-based angiogram. This test required intravenous contrast dye to "light-up" the outline of all arteries within the abdomen. The risks, besides radiation-induced cancer would be a severe allergic reaction or kidney injury. The man realized he had no choice if he wanted to find an answer to the one question clouding his mind: "Will I live or die?"

The next morning, the MRI and Angiogram test results were back. The persistent and astute doctors had finally identified a cause for the man's severe abdominal pain. Abdominal pain is often difficult to diagnose; In fact, one-third of cases of belly pain in emergency rooms never get a definite diagnosis. The severity of the pain made it crucial to find a diagnosis.

MRI result: normal. No tiny gallstones or pancreatic tumors present. A CT angiogram, however, clinched the diagnosis: A clot inside the large celiac artery due to a tear of the inner lining (dissection) of the artery. This led to reduced blood flow to the pancreas, thus causing mild damage. He could have bled to death if the artery had burst! Both of these serious conditions – the artery tearing and pancreas inflammation—cause excruciating pain. What was most remarkable about this case, aside from the excellent care the man received, was that he won that ping pong match the night his artery tore! This case is illustrative of excellent emergency room and hospital medical care for life-threatening illness. Technology and doctor sleuthing helped clarify an elusive diagnosis to properly treat serious illness, while both patient and doctors considered risks and benefits each step along the way.

Key Lessons from this True Anecdote on Handling Abdominal Pain (See also, Abdominal Pain Chapter)

1. For **severe abdominal pain** (worst ever) that prevents you from doing *any* routine daily activities, seek medical evaluation at the emergency room *immediately*. The man foolishly delayed seeking care for five days even with such severe pain. Less serious abdominal problems are likely to cause bouts of *tolerable* pain that allow the sufferer to continue routine activities, albeit with on and off discomfort.

2. **Pain and Driving Do Not Mix**: Do *not* drive yourself to an emergency room when having a severe attack of pain! The man should have called an ambulance and had his wife get his car.

3. **Chest and Abdomen Go Together**: Doctors should always consider chest problems in someone who has abdominal pain (and vice versa). Nerves in the chest and abdomen crisscross and overlap thus causing pain in more distant places removed from the actual point of origin. The ill man's doctors properly ruled out a heart attack first even though he clearly experienced abdominal pains.

4. **Avoid risky tests when possible**: The man's first imaging test was an ultrasound, not a CT scan. His doctors were correct in first

performing an ultrasound test without radiation exposure. If it identified the problem, he would have avoided that risk.

5. **Waiting for Triage**: The sick man waited about one hour in the ER waiting room before getting triaged by the nurse. He "looked pretty good" because of his high tolerance for pain. He should have spoken up and insisted he cannot wait due to severe pain and feeling weak. The desk clerk would have had a nurse immediately bring him into the main treatment area to initiate care. With pain that severe, something could have burst or ruptured during that hour of waiting, leading to death.
6. **Age Over 50 and Abdominal Pain**: As we age, that youthful, benign bellyache tends to transform into an old-age abdominal catastrophe, particularly in the elderly. Older folks more often end up having a serious abdominal problem. Moreover, seniors might not show typical outward signs of serious illness that doctors expect to see in younger adults. For instance, fever and involuntary muscle tensing are often lacking in the elderly even in the setting of a ruptured appendix. The absence of expected findings during an examination is a recipe for misdiagnosis.

II. EMERGENCY ROOM OVERCROWDING: DO NOT GET LOST IN THE CROWD

A week before Thanksgiving, 66-year-old Henry awoke in the middle of the night soaked in sweat. Chills made his teeth chatter and breathing seemed like a chore. "This flu might kill me," he mumbled to his wife.

"I will call for an appointment with the doctor," his worried wife said.

"They'll just tell me to take a fever-reducer and drink lots of water," Henry joked as he took acetaminophen and went back to bed.

The following afternoon Henry sat in the waiting room of a small medical clinic in the golden foothills of California. He felt too weak and dizzy to thumb through the stack of worn magazines near his chair. Soon a medical assistant called Henry's name and it could not have been too soon.

Henry stood up, then suddenly crashed onto the worn waiting room carpet like an aircraft falling from the sky.

"Someone call the doctor!" a man yelled out.

But the doctor had already burst through the door into the waiting room, and was kneeling by Henry's side. He was out cold, it seemed.

Vital signs: Temperature – 103 degrees, a burning fever; blood pressure – 95/55, quite low; pulse rate – 120 beats per minute, rapid; breathing rate – 26 breaths per minute and labored.

Within a minute Henry awoke. "What happened," he asked. "Why am I on the floor?"

"You are sick. I think you have an infection. Your blood pressure is so low you passed out when you stood up," the doctor explained. "In fact, you may have sepsis which is an infection that has spread to your bloodstream. You will need to be hospitalized to get antibiotics."

> An infection in people older than age 60 is serious and usually means a stay in the hospital to receive powerful antibiotics. Sepsis is more serious and may result in a much longer hospital stay.

"Ok, but an ambulance is expensive, can I call my son to drive me?" Henry asked.

"No, you have to go by ambulance," the doctor insisted. "I'm worried you might pass out before you get to the ER."

"ER? Can't you just admit me directly onto the hospital's medical floor?" asked Henry.

"You need an ER evaluation to stabilize your condition. Then one of the hospital-based doctors can admit you into the hospital," the doctor said.

> Many primary care physicians who work in an office setting no longer take care of patients when they are in the hospital. Office-based physicians and hospital-based physicians are quickly replacing the Marcus Welby doctor model of previous generations. The emergency

room has become the gateway into the hospital since lab tests, x-rays and treatments can be done quickly and around-the-clock. Specialists can be called into the ER for more complex care. Admitting doctors who care for patients after they leave the emergency room are called Hospitalists, most of whom have training in Internal Medicine.

A long line of yellow stretchers awaited Henry at the entrance door when he arrived by ambulance. A nurse screened all new patients, asking each patient a series of questions and taking vital signs. Several minutes passed before it was Henry's turn.

"So what have we here," asked a frazzled nurse.

"We picked up Mr. Barnes at his doctor's office. The doctor said he would call the emergency room to explain. His doctor thinks he has an infection," the medic explained.

"Well, no one called us," the nurse replied.

Henry's doctor actually had called the emergency room and told a physician that his patient had a blood infection and needed intravenous fluids, antibiotics and a detailed work up. But as happens too often, the rushed physician had scribbled the information on a scrap of paper then ran off to treat a critically ill patient, never relaying Henry's information.

Henry was placed inside a hallway in an open space against the wall. A nurse started an intravenous line and drew blood to be sent to the lab. While it seemed Henry was finally getting the attention he needed to begin treatment, this emergency room visit would not turn out as planned. Sadly, this is an all too common occurrence in chaotic emergency rooms worldwide.

It took some time before a doctor came in to examine Henry. The ER doctor was worried.

"I'm going to give you two different intravenous antibiotics, along with fluids. We'll take some x-rays, and I'll call the hospitalist to admit you." the hurried doctor explained. Off he went to the next sick patient.

> Hospitals are expected to meet specific time standards in the delivery of care. In Henry's case, anyone hospitalized for pneumonia must receive antibiotics within four hours of arrival. Henry had been there two hours, and rather than wait for an x-ray result in someone who almost certainly had pneumonia, the doctor ordered the antibiotics before seeing his chest x-ray.

Inside a dark hallway, between the emergency department and the main hospital, a line of eight gurneys, lined up bumper to bumper, were resting against the side wall. All were filled with sick or injured patients awaiting admission into the hospital. Henry's wife found him on one of the gurneys. It had been six hours since Henry had received his first and only dose of antibiotics.

"I'm so glad you are here," Henry whispered to his wife. "I am so thirsty, but no one will give me a glass of water. I need to go to the bathroom but can't get anybody to help me."

> Sometimes patients who are undergoing x-ray or lab testing, or who have been admitted but are awaiting an empty bed in the main hospital, are left lingering in the hallways. This is called "ER boarding of admitted patients." A lucky patient will have a nurse assigned to provide care, tend to their needs, and administer medication. But all too often there are not enough nurses to go around so hallway patients may be left for hours at a time to fend for themselves.

Mrs. Barnes tracked down a nurse and complained about her husband needing to go to the bathroom. Her complaint hit up against a brick wall: "That's not my area. You'll have to talk to the head nurse." Instead, Mrs. Barnes asked a receptionist to let her speak to the ER doctor who cared for Henry.

The ER doctor explained that Henry had pneumonia, and was

admitted to the hospital under Dr. McCormick's care, who was now the only doctor responsible for Henry. "I'm sure Dr. McCormick will see him as soon as she can," the doctor said as he sprinted off to the next crisis that just arrived through the metal ER doors.

Mrs. Barnes wondered what to do. She located a paper cup and brought her husband a glass of water. She stood by his gurney as doctors and nurses whizzed by. Soon she was told to go to the waiting room because the hallway was packed with visitors. Mrs. Barnes protested, but the ruffled nurse threatened to call security.

Ten hours after arriving in the crowded emergency room, Henry was still stuck in that overcrowded hallway. Rushed doctors and nurses flew by his gurney as if he was now just a fixture. He raised his hand to get help, but to no avail. To the ER staff in scrubs and white coats who sped by, Henry appeared like just another confused and sick old patient flailing about in a mental fog. By now, Henry felt as if a ton of bricks fell onto his chest. Each breath felt like running a marathon.

"Hey, look at that guy, he's white as a sheet!" yelled one medical student attempting to make her way through the cramped hallway.

"Let's check him out," another student said. "Hello, my name is Angie, are you okay?" she shouted into Henry's ear.

Henry did not stir. Angie shook him, but Henry did not awaken. His skin felt ice cold. Shockingly, Henry had been dead for a while. He died in the emergency room hallway while dozens of medical professionals had passed right by. The student then followed resuscitation protocol to determine if someone truly had a cardiac arrest. She shook him.

"John, go get one of the medical residents and call a code. I'll start CPR," Angie yelled with panic in her voice. Another student performed chest compressions on Henry and could feel some ribs snapping beneath. Angie tried to blow a few breaths of air into his mouth, but was repulsed by the vomit that blocked Henrys airway. People up and down the hallway gawked at the spectacle when a medical resident and intern finally arrived. "Let's get him into the resuscitation room," the resident ordered.

Henry was wheeled down the hallway back into the main emergency department where nearly a dozen health professionals pounced on him.

Some started IV lines, others mixed medications. The doctor in charge finally arrived to place a breathing tube down Henry's throat.

"All clear," yelled a voice from the crowd as the two shiny metallic paddles zapped Henry's chest with 300 Joules of electricity. Henry's limp body bounced a few inches off the stretcher.

The room was silent as everyone looked at the heart monitor. "He has a rhythm!" shouted a nurse." But the transient electrical activity from Henry's heart was typical before a stalled heart went permanently silent. Soon his heart went flat line.

The team worked on Henry for another twenty minutes, snapping more ribs and inserting more tubes and lines into a lifeless, limp body. For Henry, there was no privacy, no dignity, and no life left. The attending then officially pronounced him dead.

"Why was this guy stuck in the hallway?" the attending asked, like a coach asking his players why they lost the ballgame.

"I think the hospital shut down two wards to save money," a brave medical student replied.

"Has anyone notified next of kin?" the doctor asked. The consensus was that relatives could not be reached.

An hour later Henry's wife, who was still in the waiting room, approached the registration window. "Can you tell me if my husband has been moved upstairs into a regular hospital bed yet?"

The receptionist's eyes widened as she made a phone call. She soon looked up at the worried woman. "I'm sorry, but they tell me he passed away."

III. TRIAGE OVERSIGHTS PROVE TRAGIC

Triage Tragedy #1

George wondered if the biscuits and clam chowder he had just eaten during an executive lunch caused the sharp pain in his stomach. He regretted eating so fast as he popped a few antacid tablets. Soon the retired tradesman was doubled over in pain so he headed to the ER after his family doctor's office told him they were over-booked. His choice: A teaching hospital a few miles more distant than the local community hospital with the hope of having better access to expert specialists and around-the-clock availability of tests and treatments.

Abdominal pain can have both serious and minor causes but it can be difficult to determine which pain will go away and which will get worse. In fact, George was in good company since nearly ten percent of all emergency room visits are for this common complaint.

Once at the teaching hospital ER triage line, he stood behind mothers with crying babies, pale elderly men, and foreign laborers with injuries and various ailments. During the long wait George's abdominal pain reached a crescendo; he now felt woozy and his hearing faded slightly.

"Next!" said the triage nurse, "What can I help you with today?"

Nearly every large emergency room has a triage nurse speak to patients as they arrive. The job of the triage nurse is to rank patients based upon how sick they are. More serious illnesses get faster attention. Most nurses follow written or computer protocols, but they must exercise some judgment in their evaluation.

"My stomach hurts," George mumbled.

"How long has your stomach hurt?" she prodded.

"It started after lunch."

"Any vomiting or diarrhea?"

"No."

"Fever or chills?"

"No."

"On a scale of one to 10, with 10 the worst, how bad is your pain?" she asked.

"Seven."

"The Nurse continued to fire off many questions, not really letting George do much explaining. She took George's vital signs: BP 118/68, okay. Pulse, respiratory rate, and temperature: normal.

The triage nurse issued her decision: "Take a seat in the waiting room. We will call you when we have an empty exam room inside the department."

Minutes felt like hours as George sat slumped in his waiting room chair, his belly throbbing, head spinning, sweat percolating through his skin pores. "What else could I do?" he thought, "just follow orders." Not knowing all his options and not taking action would prove to have devastating consequences.

Two long hours passed and a tearful George could no longer bear the pain. He returned to speak to the triage nurse, who had been replaced by a young male nurse. He protested that he was feeling worse, but the busy triage nurse snapped at him to take his seat. The nurse should have known that abdominal pain in anyone over aged 50 can prove to be a catastrophic illness, and every ER should prioritize older patients with belly pain like they would a person with a heart attack.

After a few more hours of waiting, George went to use the waiting area restroom. He vomited and felt like a kid on a carousel. When he mustered enough strength he went directly to see the triage nurse again. "I feel real sick, and just vomited. How long until I can see a doctor?"

"It is pretty busy," the nurse replied. "I will call you when a room opens up. Some critically ill patients just arrived by helicopter."

"But I'm really dizzy," George protested meekly. He was too weak to argue.

"Use this plastic container if you need to vomit. If you vomit blood return immediately." The nurse handed George a shallow, curved plastic pan, like one a banana split might be served in at an ice cream parlor. George should have insisted on being evaluated by the doctor. The triage nurse also should have done a more thorough reevaluation of George, including vital signs. Some patients simply lay down on the floor near triage to get immediate medical attention. Perhaps George should have done that.

Ten hours after sitting in the hot, stuffy, noisy and crowded emergency room, the chatter of the waiting room suddenly quieted and gave way to shrieks. George crashed onto the ground with a loud thud. The woman sitting next to him yelled for help. Several attendants rushed out from behind the metallic main department doors. They quickly tossed George onto a gurney and raced him through. Doctors, nurses, and medical students surrounded him. Blood pressure: barely detectable. Breathing: too shallow to sustain life. George mumbled incoherently. Two large bore intravenous lines were jabbed into his arm veins. A narrow brown tube was passed into his bladder to monitor urine output.

The doctors had reached the big decision point: To tube him or not to tube him. The "tube" is officially called the endotracheal tube, a clear piece of plastic tubing the diameter of a narrow garden hose, but only about a foot long. This tube is passed through the mouth into the trachea or main breathing tube so a machine can pump air into the lungs. The senior ER doctor complained bitterly: "Why didn't this guy have the sense to come to the emergency room sooner? Let's tube him."

The doctors then gave him paralyzing drugs to make it easier to insert the breathing tube. George's protests eased away as his body went limp from the drugs he received. Then they shipped him off for CT scans in the nearby Radiology Department.

After hours of squirming and suffering that George experienced, and triage oversights by the triage nurses who rebuffed George's muted pleas for help, finally a diagnosis: the CT scan revealed a ruptured aortic aneurysm or swelling and leakage of the lining of the major blood vessel in the body. This tear in the major body artery allowed blood to pour out into the interior of his body. It is a true life-threatening emergency that can be treated if diagnosed and treated promptly.

But George's aortic aneurysm was not diagnosed in time. The surgeons were called to operate but George had lost too much blood. CPR had already begun. His feeble attempts to get help sooner as well as significant triage errors, combined with an overcrowded, chaotic ER proved to be the final nails in his coffin.

Triage Tragedy #2

The searing pain in Hilda's back brought tears to her eyes. She could barely hobble to the dinner table to eat a sandwich her husband had prepared. After a few days of suffering it was time to get her back checked out in the emergency room… again. The middle-aged woman spent most of the day waiting to be seen at the emergency room a couple of days ago. Hours later she was finally evaluated by a rushed doctor. After getting a back x-ray, the doctor lectured her on the need to lose weight for the back pain to improve.

Now it seemed she would again be subjected to the "blame the victim" game some doctors play. Only this trip to the ER seemed different. As she eased herself into the car, Hilda noticed her pants were moist from leaked urine. It was clear this go-round would be even more humiliating than the first visit.

Waiting ten minutes to see the triage nurse seemed like an eternity as spasms rumbled across her back. She was asked a series of questions and was told to sit in the waiting room… again.

"But I was here yesterday, why do I need to wait again?" Hilda asked.

"Because there are sicker patients ahead of you," the triage nurse replied. "And *everyone* gets back pain sooner or later."

"But I leaked urine and I'm wet," Hilda pleaded.

"Everyone at your age starts leaking urine. Get your family doctor to refer you to a urologist," the nurse said.

The events that followed that triage encounter would prove to be shocking.

Hilda pleaded with the nurse but to no avail. She trudged toward an open seat with one hand supporting her lower back, the other grabbing on to chairs or any surface to keep from collapsing.

Hour one of waiting brought more tears to her eyes as she prayed for a few moments of reprieve. Hour two brought desperation as the stabbing pain peaked. Hour three brought humiliation as more urine leaked, causing a rancid ammonia odor to waft across the waiting area. Those who sat nearby began abandoning their seats next to Hilda, trying not to be too obvious. Hilda knew why. Hour four was focused on staying seated as her body felt like melting ice cream, wanting to drip off the chair to the ground. Hour five brought severe sweats soaking her entire body. Hilda could only focus on her perspiration, worried her body odor now overwhelmed the rancid urine smell. Hour six brought a general numbness and brain haze during which she could not feel much of anything.

After six hours of eternal waiting, Hilda was finally called to pass through those metal ER doors. But there was a problem: she could not get up. It was not a matter of pain. It was not a matter of her obesity. Her legs had lost their strength. She tried again to arise and she tumbled forward, her large body thumping the floor. Emergency workers ran to her assistance and lifted her onto a stretcher. They quickly wheeled her inside, like the emergency case she had always been, only now it was too little, too late.

The doctor suspected there was compression of her spinal cord, and after another wait to get an MRI, the spinal compression diagnosis was confirmed. A neurosurgeon rushed her into the operating room for emergency surgery, but could not help her. Hilda would be paralyzed below her waist for the rest of her life.

IV. CARE NEAR THE END OF LIFE: DNR FORMS FALL SHORT

Liz had fought her way back from death's door and decided one round trip from the Pearly Gates was enough. Next time she would rather turn the doorknob and enter. Liz was blessed with more than eight decades of good health despite her smoking and drinking vices. She led an active lifestyle and kept busy with charity and other volunteer work.

Then her healthful house of cards came tumbling down. It started with cellulitis, a deep leg infection, that required hospitalization. Soon she underwent surgery on that leg. Not long after, her heart puttered out and a pacemaker was inserted. This was followed by breathing failure requiring a ventilator for a short time. Now, she recognized her memory was not what it once was.

After discussion with her family, it seemed to be an easy decision during her transition from independent living to an adult care home: she would sign a Do Not Resuscitate (DNR) form and that would address her concerns. She did not want to endure another round of medical calamity, painful procedures and intensive care despair. She believed her time should have been up on the first go-round.

Liz's presumed "easy" DNR decision, however, turned into an in-depth discussion with family and serious soul-searching, as well as heavy life-and-death discussions that are best pondered over many years, not days.

Signing a DNR form, the doctor explained, was not nearly sufficient to be secure in a "happy death" and better quality of life during her remaining time.

All the DNR form does, her doctor emphasized, was tell healthcare workers not to do chest compressions or insert a breathing tube if her heart or breathing suddenly stopped, meaning she would have *died.* DNR addresses the event of death only (breathing or heart stoppage), but says nothing of her wishes in the gray zone during her remaining months to years of life. What if she developed pneumonia which compromised her breathing? If she deteriorated would she want a breathing tube inserted for a few days with the hope her pneumonia would resolve and breathing status would also improve? If she became dehydrated or suffered a serious but treatable acute illness, would she want to go to the hospital for a short course of aggressive treatment? What would be her wishes if she became non-communicative or comatose? Would she want her pacemaker turned off near the end of life so it does not prolong an imminent death? Is a feeding tube an option if she loses the ability to take in nutrition the old fashioned way? How about intravenous fluids? At what point, if any, would Liz want to undergo or forego kidney dialysis if her kidneys went kaput? What would be Liz's red line for refusing unexpected surgery such as a gallbladder attack during her remaining months of life? Liz could simply assign a preferred healthcare proxy (substitute decision maker) and hope that person makes all the right decisions. That is asking for a lot, however, even if the proxy has her best intentions at heart. A great deal of emotion, confusion and uncertainty enters into these choices, including guilt that not doing everything is tantamount to accelerating a loved one's death. Detailed instructions with clearly stated quality-of-life red lines can unburden family members.

The deep discussion for a happy death does not end with a list of procedures Liz would or would not wish to have at specific points in her health decline. The more difficult work is defining those quality-of-life red lines, beyond which Liz would want only basic comfort measures for pain and suffering. Is that red line an irreversible coma? Loss of ability to recognize or communicate with loved ones? Perhaps being bedridden and fully dependent on others is an unfathomable situation for her? Inability to do treasured activities such as look at family photos or read art books or laugh with grandchildren during visits might be a defining loss that triggers a decision of no further interventions. These philosophical decisions are intensely personal. Nobody else can pinch hit for you and accurately draw subtle red lines for your own "happy death" or quality of life. Equally important is the task of finding life meaning and contentment. Mending broken relationships and expressing feelings to valued friends and loved ones during your final months or years is also priceless.

When Liz signed that DNR form, it proved to be only the beginning of her "die-happy" planning, not the final step as she had expected.

V. WRONG DIAGNOSIS: TOO MUCH TRUST IN IMPERFECT TESTS

As if a bad cough and cold were not enough, 46-year-old Veronica woke her husband up during the night complaining of unfamiliar chest pains that seemed to travel to her shoulder blades and arms. These were strange symptoms for a health-conscious and active woman with a resting heart rate low enough to make any athlete blush. A trip to an urgent care center took four hours to find out she had a relatively normal electrocardiogram and chest x-ray, but definitely abnormal blood enzyme levels that clearly signaled heart damage. Nitroglycerin and aspirin were administered before she was high-tailed out of urgent care by ambulance. Destination: nearest emergency department.

Both the emergency room doctor and cardiologist at the community hospital confidently explained to Veronica that she suffered a mild heart attack and needed an angiogram to evaluate the condition of her heart-feeding arteries. Turns out, her arteries were normal and clean as a whistle.

Veronica's chest discomfort persisted so she spent the next couple of days in an intensive care unit with monitors beeping incessantly and all-day awakenings and interruptions. If the disease won't kill the patient, she wondered, the care might.

With "good behavior" and improvement in her condition, Veronica was released from the hospital to follow up with a university hospital internist. It took a couple of weeks to get in to see that doctor. What that internist told her would shatter all her closely-held beliefs about those few daunting days of sickness and pain.

The day of her visit to follow up with an internist at a nearby university hospital, Veronica continued to experience shortness of breath climbing stairs and required many extra hours of sleep each day. Would she now be a cardiac invalid? Yet the angiogram did not find any major heart disease or damage – were those doctors wrong?

The internist reviewed all her hospital records, took a careful history of her illness experience, and repeated an electrocardiogram. After discussion with experienced colleagues, the internist rocked her world.

"You *didn't* have a heart attack," he said calmly and confidently.

Veronica and her husband were shocked. One set of doctors was surely mistaken. Which one was it?

A university cardiologist performed an echocardiogram (ultrasound of the heart) and confirmed the true diagnosis: there was evidence of mild heart-pumping inefficiency. The diagnosis: myocarditis, an inflammation of the heart muscle caused by the respiratory virus she and her children contracted before all the chaos began. Those community hospital and urgent care doctors jumped to a conclusion of heart attack based upon a blood test known to confirm heart muscle damage. However, there are several possible causes for damage to heart muscle besides a clot in a heart-feeding artery (heart attack). No heart damage was detectable on the angiogram. A relatively normal initial electrocardiogram and no risk factors at all for coronary artery disease in a relatively young woman were all clues something was amiss. It seemed the abnormal heart enzyme blood test called Troponin misled those who always believed in it.

This story is a summary of a true case report based upon an essay written by Veronica's husband, Harold Pollack, and published in the *American Prospect* in 2008.

VI. 911 AMBULANCE TRAUMA SYSTEM: TOO MUCH OF A GOOD THING?

A passerby noticed sixty-four-year-old Sam Holmes lying on the ground near his bicycle at the foot of a massive oak tree. Sam appeared unconscious so the concerned citizen dialed 911: "I found a bicyclist who crashed his bike against a tree and is out cold. I think you better send an ambulance here." The man relayed the location then rushed off to his destination.

Several minutes later an ambulance arrived, lights and sirens frightening away nearby birds and squirrels. The senior paramedic jumped out of the ambulance and ran over to Mr. Holmes. "What happened?" she asked as she shook his shoulder and rubbed his chest.

Holmes could only moan and mumble a few words. The paramedic could not understand what he said.

The paramedic reassured Mr. Holmes. "Don't worry, we'll take care of you. Just be still."

A junior paramedic had already brought a long plastic board from the ambulance, and was at his partner's side. "Let's get a cervical collar on his neck first. I'm worried about a spine injury," said the more experienced paramedic. "Then we can carefully strap him to the backboard."

The junior paramedic noticed Mr. Holmes' wallet and a scrap of paper resting on the ground beside his still body, but there was no time to lose focus. The medic stuffed the paper and wallet into Mr. Holmes' pocket and they strapped him to the backboard, as is standard protocol. Mr. Holmes was soon gasping for air because the collar felt like a boot pressing on his neck.

"Should we intubate him," the junior medic asked?

"No, I think he is getting enough air," the senior paramedic replied as she listened with her stethoscope to Mr. Holmes' lungs. "Let's just get him right to the ER," she said.

They scooped up the sick man and slid him into the ambulance. Once inside, following protocol, they decided to start an intravenous line — a tube that would deliver salt water into his veins to help support weak circulation in case he lost a lot of blood internally. By appearances, he had no signs of bleeding.

It took several minutes to start the intravenous line. The medics then called headquarters and requested permission to take Mr. Holmes, an apparent bicycle accident victim, to the regional trauma center located thirty miles away, rather than the nearest local hospital. The dispatcher replied: "The interstate is jammed up, so I'll call the helicopter to meet you at the nearest fire station, about four miles east of your location." The dispatcher gave the exact location, and within minutes the helicopter reached an open field next to the fire station and swooped down into the open landing zone.

The senior paramedic gave the flight nurse report: "Sixty-four-year-old male who appears to have crashed his bike into a tree – unwitnessed and unknown speed. Reduced level of alertness. Probable head trauma, his helmet was a few feet away. Blood pressure 80 with weak, thready pulse. We have him on a spine board and started an IV. He has gotten about half a bag."

The helicopter nurse then loaded the patient aboard a B-117 chopper, one of the best medical transport flying machines. As the experienced flight nurse tended to him, she wondered why he had no scrapes, bruises or broken bones after flying off a bicycle.

Fifteen minutes later they reached the rooftop of the regional trauma center, and unloaded Mr. Holmes, who was asking in a confused voice, "What happened? Where am I?"

The patient was wheeled into the ER trauma resuscitation room where several surgery training-program doctors and a few nurses waited. They had received a report of a bike crash victim with dangerously low blood pressure. Without saying a word, workers snipped off the man's clothes and inserted another intravenous line into his arm. Mr. Holmes protested and tried to push away trespassing hands. He then mumbled "Where am I? Where's my wife? Is she here yet?"

The senior surgery resident explained: "He is obviously confused and uncooperative, probably from his head injury. He has a red spot on his forehead – maybe a bruise. Let's just intubate him and flood him with two liters of IV saline (salt water). Let's get his pressure up guys."

The residents then gave Mr. Holmes paralyzing and sedating drugs to induce a hazy slumber. They placed a plastic breathing tube through his mouth into his trachea – the main breathing passage. He was then hooked up to a ventilator machine and tubes of blood were sent for testing and blood-type matching. Two liters of saline poured into his veins with little change in blood pressure, then four more bags of salt-water ultimately flooded his circulation system. The man was whisked off to the Radiology department where he underwent CT scans of his head, neck, chest, and abdomen. By then he had received seven liters of salt water in his body, into a blood system with limited capacity beyond the usual five quarts of blood.

CT scans were completed and showed no abnormalities. The nurse caring for Mr. Holmes interrupted the residents: "His pulse ox reading is down to 85 percent oxygen level. Do you want me to turn up the O2 flow?" she asked.

"Yes… maybe he has a lung contusion (bruise) that we cannot yet see on CT scan." the resident replied.

Over the next hour, Mr. Holmes' blood oxygen levels continued to drop, meaning he was not getting enough blood and oxygen to feed vital organs. Soon the heart monitor showed irregular beats, a sign his heart was oxygen-starved. The senior resident had called the senior surgeon to review the case. "I think you are dealing with shock lung. He won't last long. Better notify next of kin," the surgeon warned.

Mr. Holmes died in the emergency room nine hours after his arrival. The actual cause of death was because his lungs had been flooded with unnecessary intravenous salt-water given by young doctors. By now, pieces of the puzzle were fitting together – only too late to save Mr. Holmes. That red spot on his forehead was not a bruise, rather it was red and swollen and resembled a hornet sting. That piece of paper that the medic hurriedly shoved into Mr. Holmes pocket – his wife found the note and read it:

> "My name's Sam Holmes. Stung by bee... feel dizzy, trouble breathing. Call wife at this number. Bring bee sting kit left at home..."

Tragically, he died after suffering a fully treatable illness – a serious allergic reaction — because of overtreatment and misdiagnosis. Emergency workers ignored the obvious *lack* of bruises and other injuries that would be present if he really suffered from a serious bicycle accident. Some emergency workers might argue Mr. Holmes should have worn a Medic Alert bracelet for his serious bee-sting allergy. Perhaps so, but if he had such a bracelet, he might have left it at home after showering since he also forgot to bring his sting kit. Emergency professionals, however, must consider all clues that point both toward or *away from* a specific diagnosis.

A few weeks later, Mrs. Holmes was shocked when she received bills totaling $69,000. The breakdown: $52,000 from the emergency room, $15,000 for the helicopter, and an ambulance bill for $2,000. A bee sting kit costs only a few dollars and was the only treatment he needed. To make matters worse, Mr. Holmes was uninsured. He had cancelled his expensive medical insurance on his 64th birthday, expecting to soon reach the Medicare-eligible age of 65. Mrs. Holmes realized she would have to sell her home and move in with her daughter.

Key Teaching Points:

- Be prepared like a boy scout. Carry a bee sting kit if allergic; carry sugar cubes with you if diabetic. Use an emergency notification system and keep it nearby if you are frail.
- Wear a **Medic Alert** bracelet if you have potentially life-threatening ailments or allergies. At a minimum, place a laminated card in your wallet or purse listing your serious ailments. In this specific case, however, neither medics nor hospital professionals checked his wallet.
- Carry a cell phone, especially if you go out alone.
- 911 systems follow protocols which might not recognize less common or serious ailments. Too much care, as well as too little, can have disastrous results.
- Trauma centers follow protocols, and might not pay close enough attention to clues and to the patient's specific details and medical history. Once a false assumption is propagated it may grow wings; clues that suggest otherwise might then be ignored or minimized. This is why the best medicine is to be prepared! Prevention and avoiding these vulnerable care situations is safest.

- Doctors and other medical professionals do not listen to patients enough. Communication is lacking. Rather than sedating Mr. Holmes into unconsciousness, perhaps the newbie young doctor should have further questioned the man and tried to make sense of his "babbling."
- The chaos and rushed approach to emergency department care can be dangerous and deadly to folks. As patient, always err on the side of caution. Be proactive. Ask questions. Insist on explanations before undergoing tests and treatments. If you are alone and unable to communicate, you can only hope for the best.
- Always remain covered by medical insurance no matter how healthy you are, especially if over 50 years of age.

SECTION IV
EMERGENCY ROOM AND HOSPITAL DANGERS (AND SOLUTIONS)

DANGER 1. EMERGENCY ROOM OVERCROWDING: SHAKING THE SODA BOTTLE

The flood of patients pouring into overcrowded emergency rooms is like shaking a soda bottle: one never knows how badly things will erupt. Overcrowding and the shaken-soda-bottle pressure that builds up have caused concern in countries around the globe. There are several different faces to overcrowding but the final appearance remains the same: reduced quality of care. Overcrowding can be hazardous to your health. The following anecdotes expose the different looks of ER overcrowding – and they are not too pretty.

Lucky Liz

Liz thought she must have slept in an awkward position when she awoke with a sharp pain in her upper back. When the pain persisted, she took a common pain reliever. No change. Hot shower: no help. Time was not kind to her as the pain increased in intensity. When Liz became aware that each breath seemed like a small chore, she sought medical care at a trusted community urgent care practice in a big city. The woman was calm and comfortable on arrival, appearing younger than her stated age of sixty. A check of vital signs revealed a soaring blood pressure. Perhaps the pressure was high because of her back pain, the doctor wondered. The experienced physician was puzzled since Liz seemed more likely to ignore ailments rather than baby them. Yet, she sought help for back pain without even a clear injury. It just did not add up. On a clinical judgment hunch that doctors often depend upon, he ordered an electrocardiogram. The squiggly lines zigged when they should have zagged. It was clearly abnormal, but not definitive for a heart attack. Liz was reluctant to go to the hospital, having difficulty believing she might be experiencing a heart problem. After all, she took care of herself and exercised regularly. After some coaxing, Liz was promptly transferred by ambulance to a nearby, busy emergency room.

Before being shipped off, the doctor wrote out a note summarizing concerns with a presumptive diagnosis of "Angina, rule out myocardial infarction." A copy of the abnormal EKG was attached, along with a verbal warning to Liz not to allow emergency staff to rush her out of the hospital. By appearances, Liz seemed a picture of health. She was neither gasping for air nor writhing in pain. Her skin color was not suntan-bronze nor was it grayish-blue. She appeared mostly calm and in no distress, perhaps a reflection of her denial more than her stoicism. Appearances sure can be deceiving. Her healthy appearance combined with her less typical symptoms of a heart problem were a setup for emergency room error and folly. Surely, the doctor's note and EKG that accompanied her would help avoid this dilemma.

A short time later, however, a doctor-in-training from the ER called the urgent care office asking for Liz's contact information. *How odd!* The doctor thought. She had just left for the hospital a couple hours earlier. *Maybe she never went to the hospital?* The doctor feared.

As things turned out, Liz was discharged from the ER within three hours, despite the urgent care doctor's admonitions. The ER was quite chaotic. Inexperienced and unsupervised doctors in training dropped the ball. They never saw the note or EKG sent with Liz. Perhaps she was too overwhelmed to mention it or was simply ignored. And they rushed her out before the heart muscle damage blood test result was back (testing took longer back then). She did, in fact, suffer a minor heart attack without a hint of chest pain. Liz was lucky since she suffered no negative events despite mistakenly being sent home. She made a full recovery.

Deck the Halls with Squirming Patients

Ronald Collins arrived at the emergency room with a really bad stomach-ache. The elderly, retired machinist was surprised when the triage nurse told him to wait in the waiting room until a physician could see him. It seemed like a zoo inside the waiting area. He pleaded for something to relieve his pain, and just as his request was refused with a stern, "Not until the doctor sees you," he vomited onto the tile waiting room floor. His wife asked for faster entry into the ER and the nurse relented.

The triage nurse brought Ronald into the ER, but instead of going to the main treatment area, he was taken into a busy hallway and led onto the only unoccupied gurney. His wife was sent back out to the waiting area to limit the number of bodies inside the patient areas.

Ronald squirmed and writhed in agony for over an hour, waving his hand for attention. He was ignored. Finally a young nurse came to take his vital signs. He complained of pain, but was told to hold out until the doctor arrives. Ronald's mouth was parched. His tongue stuck to the roof of his mouth. Yet no one would give him a drink. His belly throbbed in predictable patterns like ocean waves crashing onto rocks. Finally, a rushed doctor came to assess him. Ronald felt embarrassed that the doctor undid his clothes to examine him in front of dozens of people who walked by. The doctor promised pain medicine, an intravenous fluid drip, as well as blood tests and x-ray imaging. An hour passed and the only thing that came back was the pain. No testing. No intravenous fluids. No pain medication to numb the waves of agony. Ronald needed to use the bathroom but was too weak to walk down the hall. "Help! Help! Help me please!" he yelled.

Could this suffering and neglect have been avoided? The hospital could have staffed the department with more nurses and doctors, to be sure, but that would cost gobs of money that is simply not available. Those eight patients who decked the halls awaiting admission into the hospital should have been sent up to the wards so nurses and doctors could have paid more attention to the newly sick folks who arrived. The ER rumbling on the "chaos-Richter scale" would surely have dropped a notch or two with fewer "boarded" patients awaiting transfer into the main hospital. In a perfect ER world, Ronald would not have suffered so long and his life would not have been needlessly imperiled with delays in caring for serious abdominal pain. A definite diagnosis was never found.

Delays are dangerous in ER hallways and in the main department, but can be equally catastrophic for patients who remain unchecked in the waiting room. Consider these disturbing media headlines that convey care catastrophes from overcrowding and neglect in America's chaotic emergency departments:

Man Dies after Waiting Hours for ER to Treat His Rash

Woman Dies in ER Lobby as 911 Refuses to Help

Tape Shows Woman Dying on Waiting Room Floor

Woman with Asthma Attack Dies in Hospital Waiting Room

Texas Man Dies after Waiting 16 Hours for Treatment in ER

Emergency Room Overcrowding

Has emergency room and hospital care reached a boiling point? A point of no return? The expectation people may have had for "red-carpet" treatment for serious illness when visiting an emergency room has become a faded memory. No longer can you arrive and expect to see an empty waiting room, a smiling nurse at triage, and a doctor sitting idly, eager to treat your sudden gasping or to sew up your bloody finger.

Fifty years ago, if you walked into an emergency room chances were good that you would receive express service. As a child in the 1960's, this author (RD) experienced such care. Seeing this care model, I decided to become an emergency room physician. I expected to sit and read journals, waiting for the next patient to arrive. "Those ER doctors are like firemen, waiting to extinguish the next medical fire," my dad would tell me. After 27 years of schooling and residency training, my dream was realized. But things have surely changed.

Emergency departments have become chaotic and overcrowded in urban, suburban and even rural hospitals in the United States and abroad. This means it will take longer for you to be seen by a doctor, especially if you have what are considered less serious ailments such as cold, flu, cough, sprains or minor cuts. ER waiting rooms can surely make for a scary first impression. Crowded, noisy, smelly waiting rooms can be stuffed with dozens of people wanting for care – coughing, moaning, crying and bleeding. Waits are usually many hours to see a doctor or other healthcare provider.

But what if you suffer from a more serious problem? Abdominal pain, for instance, should be considered a medical emergency. Hospital policy (and federal law) dictates that you must be seen quickly. But your condition might not be appreciated at triage (see also, Triage Travesty chapter), and you might be forced to wait hours to see a physician. Treatment is provided on a priority, not first-come, basis. In addition, you might wait several hours while you undergo a variety of tests such as blood draws, EKGs, x-rays, CT scans and MRIs. Waiting for consultant specialists to arrive can tack on a few more hours. If you need hospital admission and are unlucky, you might be stuck in a dimly lit hallway for another 12 to 24 hours. This is known as "patient boarding."

Fast forward to the present. I *am* now that ER doctor. I don't have time to read journals nor to guzzle down a cup of coffee. At times I don't even have a minute to use the bathroom during my 12-hour work shifts. What happened?

ER Chaos and Crowds: What Gives?

Reasons for ER overcrowding are many, and cannot be blamed on any single problem, or solved with one simple solution like hiring more emergency room doctors. What exactly is emergency department overcrowding? Crowded means crowded – like a crowded airport lobby, a shopping center packed wall to wall with Christmas shoppers, or a sandy beach spotted with sunbathers on a warm Florida day. Another way to define overcrowding: When nurses and doctors feel rushed to the point that they believe quality of care is compromised.

The following list offers the most commonly cited explanations for the United States (and worldwide) emergency room overcrowding crisis. This chaos problem is not simply an academic curiosity. Each day, in every town, ER crowding and chaos harm folks who seek medical care.

1. **Patient tidal wave, more ER closures:** According to the Centers for Disease Control and Prevention, there are about 136 million emergency room visits each year, and this number continues to

climb. The number of hospital emergency rooms, however, has decreased from nearly 8,000 prior to 1990 to about 5,000 today. At the same time, the United States population has increased by more than 50 million people during the past two decades. This amounts to packing more sardines into fewer cans, so to speak.

2. **Full hospital beds:** In the distant past, it was not uncommon for hospitals to run at 50 percent occupancy. The intent was to maintain empty beds in case of a flu epidemic, natural disaster, or war. Nowadays most hospitals are overflowing. Sick or injured emergency patients are bottlenecked in ER hallways because no inpatient beds are available. These admitted patients remain in ER corridors, holding areas, and even key treatment rooms just occupying scarce space. New patient arrivals are forced to wait.

   It is more concerning that emergency rooms are not properly staffed to care for boarded patients, so both doctors and nurses must split their precious time and attention among boarded patients and sick new arrivals. These new arrivals, in turn, get slower, less focused service. The whole system can grind to a halt when critically ill patients arrive. Meanwhile, those boarded patients who deck the halls are overlooked and ignored. Should they deteriorate, patients might well die right on that stretcher in that hallway! It might take hours for someone to notice their cold, pale body and unusual silence.

3. **Time-consuming technology:** Patients, ER doctors, consulting doctors, and admitting doctors all demand more testing, treating and imaging. When I began emergency medicine practice, CT scans did not exist. If I was really worried about a head injury, I would just admit the patient into one of many open hospital beds for observation. Now head CT scans are done as part of a standard work up for minor headaches or bumps and bruises. I just check off the box on the order sheet, and then rush to the next patient. But these imaging studies take time, particularly more specialized MRIs and such. Some neurology consultants will not even come to the ER to evaluate a patient until a brain MRI has been

completed. There may be a line of patients awaiting this type of test, adding hours of waiting time for each patient.

4. **Medical malpractice fears** (see also, Malpractice chapter)**:** The availability of newfangled lab tests and fancy imaging studies creates a second set of problems: ordering studies simply as defensive medicine. Consider a 20-year-old college student with lower abdominal pain. He might look well and I am confident I can safely send him home. There is, however, a one in ten thousand risk that he has appendicitis. I can explain to him his risks and send him home with instructions to return if he gets worse. Alternatively, I can order a CT scan to exclude appendicitis, sleep better myself, and not worry about being sued. More and more CT scans are being ordered for this reason, taking up more valuable ER resources and time.

5. **More complex diseases in an aging population:** Many diagnostic tests and treatments for chronic medical diseases did not exist a generation ago. Their use now swallows up a large chunk of precious time in emergency departments. There are new and chronic diseases that require much time and energy investment to properly care for these patients in an emergency setting. Examples include HIV-related ailments, liver failure from hepatitis C, skyrocketing drug abuse, diabetes complications, dementia-related care, longer-living heart failure and emphysema patients, and adverse reactions to medications and risky therapies. New treatments for cancer have saved or prolonged many lives, yet these treatments are tainted by serious side effects and complications requiring emergency care. Kidney dialysis patients are now frequent fliers in our nation's emergency rooms. Some people with serious diseases have their lives extended another decade because of miracle medicines and technology. But one of the costs of those added years may be multiple trips to the ER during flare-ups of illness or from complications of treatment.

6. **Primary care office overflow:** The old model of comprehensive care by your primary care doctor is rapidly changing. In the past, most primary care doctors took care of their patients both in the

office for minor problems, and in the hospital if their patients needed advanced care. The doctor would call the admissions office and arrange for a sick patient to be admitted. The doctor would phone in treatment orders to the floor nursing station. If you got sick at night or on weekends and called your doctor, he or she would make admission arrangements by phone. Each morning, and often in the evening, the doctor would go to the hospital, examine their hospitalized patients, do procedures, and revise orders. But care processes have changed. Primary care doctors are pressured into seeing 50 office patients each day to keep up with high practice costs. They have no time to add on urgencies. There is also little incentive to see urgencies since payment is not high enough to warrant squeezing in extra patients who might be quite sick and time-consuming. Liability worries dictate that the moderately sick patient who calls for an appointment will be directed to the ER since a delay of a day or two (if that quick an appointment is even possible) might allow the patient to deteriorate, thus leading to lawsuits – even if the illness did not seem life-threatening. What's more, covering on-call doctors in a practice will quickly refer unfamiliar, moderately sick patients to an emergency room rather than undertake liability risk and tell the patient to wait until the next day to be seen in the office.

7. **Leaving without being seen**: It is common for patients to leave a crowded ER without ever getting a doctor evaluation when waits take too long. One in 20 of these folks who leave an ER will require hospitalization within two weeks, according to a past study of this problem. They often wind up at another emergency room.
8. **Other factors causing overcrowding**: These include a flood of mental illness patients in crisis; delays as emergency departments now use electronic medical records that can require giving more attention to the computer than to the patients; doctor and nurse understaffing due to tight budget constraints; high rate of burnout and turnover amongst nurses and doctors in this chaotic setting, causing the best and most experienced care providers to be replaced by novices.

In summary, the subject of ER overcrowding is more than academic, with the following real potential consequences for patients:

- Longer waits and stays have become routine and expected.
- Ambulance diversion of seriously ill patients to more distant hospitals can cause delays in receiving critical care.
- Higher death rate. For instance, chest pain sufferers who went to an *overcrowded* ER had three times greater risk for bad outcomes such as heart failure and cardiac arrest, according to a July 2009 study in *Academic Emergency Medicine.*
- Risk of becoming a "boarded" patient: as you deck the halls for hours to days awaiting a hospital inpatient bed, your care suffers. You get limited monitoring and oversight as you are placed in "care purgatory." ER staff and inpatient doctors and nurses may point their finger in the other direction if you ask who is responsible for your care while boarded in a hallway or holding area.
- Misdiagnosed serious illness and careless treatment are real risks. Errors in care are more likely to occur after midnight or during times of extreme chaos and overcrowding. Be sure to always request that the most experienced doctor in charge evaluates you before you are discharged or admitted whenever serious illness is at stake.
- False reassurance that all is okay is a danger when a cursory evaluation is done. Perhaps one test is performed to exclude a disease that is unrelated to your actual problem as the ER doctor barks up the wrong tree. All this in the interest of rushing to get you out of the crowded department.
- Medication errors are ever-present risks.
- Important test results may not be checked or confirmed as correctly interpreted by a more experienced doctor or specialist.
- One can experience treatment delays for serious illnesses such as heart attack or pneumonia that require prompt start of treatment for best outcomes.
- Avoidable suffering, discomfort and loss of dignity are too common.

- Avoidable spread of infections like flu or other viruses, measles and tuberculosis in crowded waiting rooms or emergency department hallways are real risks.
- The sleepy doctor: Up to 24-hour shifts can cause fatigue and mental strain in ER doctors and nurses. The result: more errors in care.

Solutions to Avoid Overcrowded Emergency Rooms and Sub-Par Care

What could go wrong when well-trained professionals stretch the boundaries of dedication to care for seriously sick folks? Quite a lot. There are no accurate statistics tallied on patient harm, death and suffering that might have been avoided with more focused and prompt care. Subtle harm, neglect and oversights oft go unnoticed and unmentioned. The simple answer is to avoid the ER whenever possible; but that is not always an option. The goal is to use emergency rooms only for potentially life-threatening illness. Following are some helpful suggestions:

1. Discover through recommendations and research the locations of nearby community hospital and urgent care facilities with quality reputations. For common variety illnesses and injuries, these smaller hospitals and walk-in practices are excellent alternatives to the high cost, high chaos and long waits of busier teaching or university hospital emergency rooms.
2. Just a reminder: Ideally, common variety ailments should be tended to by a family doctor. A good relationship with a trusted primary care doctor or nurse practitioner can prove invaluable for better care and urgent attention on short notice.
3. Timing is everything, they say. So true. If an emergency room trip is necessary, the worst times in most ERs to pay a visit are Mondays, all day; and Friday nights and Saturday nights. During flu season better stay away unless your life depends upon it. If you were not too sick on arrival, you may well catch something bad during cold and flu season. The best of times: Early mornings tend to be slower times. Many emergency rooms now have online wait time estimates. Be cautious with checking those because it can be slow when you start your car and chaotic a half-hour later when

two heart attack victims and a three-car pileup add some spice to the quiet morning. Another admonition: Never use the word "quiet" when in the ER. Staff will accuse you of jinxing them when treatment rooms quickly (and inevitably, of course) start filling up.

4. Consider trying a freestanding emergency department (FED) for care. These facilities, physically separate from hospitals, are equipped to treat more serious illness than can urgent care. They are usually staffed by emergency medicine-certified doctors. It is estimated that more than two-thirds of ER visits nationally could be managed outside the hospital emergency room setting, according to the Centers for Disease Control and Prevention. FEDs also tend to be less busy than standard emergency rooms. The disadvantages: Limited availability in more upscale neighborhoods in states such as Texas, California, Florida and Colorado. As many as 40 states now boast offering at least a few FEDs. Costs at these facilities can be triple that of an urgent care center. These facilities mostly do *not* accept Medicare or Medicaid insurance.

5. Another alternative to rushing immediately to an ER for less serious illness is to first call a nurse helpline service provided by your health insurer. Sometimes simple, common sense advice and tincture of time can allow health problems to resolve naturally.

6. At times, calling an ambulance can be the solution. Paramedics or experienced emergency medical technicians might evaluate you for a quickly-resolving ailment and find you are much improved with normal vitals. An EKG tracing to evaluate the heart may also be done. If all is good, you might simply arrange an appointment with your family doctor rather than seeking immediate ER transport.

7. Do not be enticed by advertisements guaranteeing prompt ER evaluation in less than 30 minutes, for instance. First, those numbers are fudged by getting a doctor to do a lightning-fast eyeball evaluation and say hello, then you sit and wait. Second, you would not want ER doctors rushing your care to beat the clock. Some of these advertised emergency departments, however, are better organized and more efficient.

8. If you are having a bad emergency room care experience, you can

contact the hospital patient representative or an administrator to get some support. For instance, if you are being sent home but feel quite ill and believe you should get observation or further evaluation a patient rep can prove to be helpful. A complaint letter sent to the hospital administrator, state Department of Health, and your health insurer using an old-fashioned postal letter might be worthwhile. You can also share your ER story – good or bad – on the BoomER-Survival Guide website. (see Bulk Purchase page, back of book).

9. Beware the "Sloppy Joe" physician. Some Physicians are lazy and care more about their stock investments than you. They will take short cuts to get patients out of the ER, either by premature discharges to home or inappropriate admissions into the hospital. How can you identify a "Sloppy Joe" doctor? These doctors may spend fleeting moments at your bedside, offer few explanations about your status and little reassurance and hope. They may order many tests without first explaining the pros and cons, nor getting your input in decision-making.

DANGER 2. TRIAGE TRAVESTY: DANGERS OF CHECKING-IN AT AN EMERGENCY ROOM

Checking into an emergency room for care seems like a straightforward process. You describe your problem, reel off some personal demographic information, flash your health insurance card, then you are good to go. You are now in the queue to be seen soon. Well, not so fast. Triage is far more important and complex than simply "signing into" the emergency room or urgent care facility. This medical care screening process is nothing like taking a ticket number when waiting at the deli, bakery or motor vehicle department. Proper triage actually can determine your fate. When done poorly, triage can doom you to long waits, poor quality care or even death!

When checking in for care, you do not get evaluated on a first come, first serve basis. The concept of triage was imported from France, it is believed, from the battlefields of the First World War. Translated, "triage" means "to sort." On the battlefield, medics sorted through the many injured soldiers to identify those who needed immediate care for survival and those who could no longer be helped.

Consider the well-publicized travesty of triage that happened in Texas several years back, as detailed in a 2011 *The Dallas Morning News* article. Following is a summary of events described in that article:

A 58-year-old man trudged into a busy Dallas, Texas emergency room complaining of severe abdominal pain. Perhaps he was stoic and did not appear too distressed because the triage nurse assigned his complaint a level 3 urgency — care within 60 minutes. This middle ranking on the five-level triage system used by most emergency rooms is commonly used for those suffering with abdominal pain. This is a huge mistake and must be changed! Abdominal pain, particularly in those over age 50, is frequently a symptom of life-threatening illness. For this middle aged man in Texas, his family had to learn this the hard way.

The triage nurse took his vital signs, documented that he said his abdominal pain was a "10," the highest pain level, and told the man to wait in the waiting room. Appearances can be deceiving: Those who have high pain tolerance can appear okay despite looming disaster.

Incredibly, a woman sitting next to this sick man in the waiting room noticed his distress and began to pressure nurses to get him evaluated. She was rebuffed by the staff. She even called her father and told him the man next to her was going to die, according to the article.

The hour hand on the clock traveled quite a distance and the sun rose many hours later before this man was called in for evaluation. The doctor who evaluated him, it turns out, was a novice doctor-in-training who had just completed medical school. There is no substitute for experienced eyes in cutting through the chaos and recognizing looming crisis in someone who is subtly but seriously ill. The young doctor lacked those experienced eyes when he ordered some tests and a pain pill. The man soon vomited up the medication, collapsed onto the stretcher and died, before an intravenous line could be inserted.

The coroner attributed his death to heart disease. Perhaps that abdominal pain, as it turned out, was a less typical manifestation of a heart attack in progress? The man had a known history of heart problems that never came up during the brief triage interview – a crucial error, to be sure. One cannot imagine the suffering he experienced during 17 hours of writhing abdominal distress. There was also an apparent lack of proper reassessment of a truly ill waiting-room patient as required by emergency room policy.

There is an art and science to the process of triage. In the United States, usually a registered nurse will do a quick interview with you, "eyeball" your appearance, and assess your vital signs. Depending on how busy it is, the nurse has about a minute or two. Urgent care facilities may well screen you with an untrained front-desk assistant who will call for help if you appear real sick. Most emergency rooms now use computer software triage systems to determine one of five levels of severity of your illness or injury: Immediate (under one minute to evaluate), emergent (under 14 minutes), urgent (under 60 minutes), semi-urgent (under two hours), non-urgent (within 24 hours to evaluate). There is some evidence these software algorithms for emergency care are not very accurate; in truth, they fall apart when it comes to older adults and frail elderly. Older folks usually have less typical signs and symptoms of disease and may provide less than accurate details of an illness. Many old folks have communication difficulty due to memory loss, hearing loss and speech deficits. This leads to inaccurate or limited guidance in formulating a most likely diagnosis or two. The elderly often are sicker than they look when they enter an emergency room. For example, abdominal pain is often assigned a mid-range urgency category (under 60 minutes) despite high risk for life-threatening illness in adults over age 50 who are experiencing belly pain. Seniors with this complaint have a ten-fold higher risk for serious illness than younger adults, and often require surgery. Sixty minutes of wait time (level III priority) can easily turn into a few hours during times of ER chaos. In an ideal system, abdominal pain *should be* considered level I or II priority until proven not to be life threatening.

The following anecdote is another example of how serious illness can be masked as minor complaints — a wolf-like disease in sheep's clothing, so to speak.

A man leaned on the registration desk of a city emergency room and in heavily accented English asked for help. With his two young children at his side, he explained to the person seated at the sign-in desk how he had awakened three hours earlier from sleep with sharp shoulder pain.

"Which shoulder hurts?" the woman asked.

"My left," he mumbled, as he grimaced and clutched his shoulder.

"Did you fall, sir?" She looked up at his pale face.

"No, no. When I woke up," he repeated. By now he used the desk to help support his weight.

His printed chart read: "Chief complaint, left shoulder pain x three hours." The triage nurse stuffed his chart under a thick pile of patient charts yet to be called. After all, it was just an orthopedic problem. In the waiting room, the man steadied his spinning head between his hands. Soon a soaking sweat drenched him. While his children were giggling at magazine pictures, the man suddenly slid onto the floor, shocking others waiting for care. His children paced around the room pleading for help as their father's eyes bulged out, teeth clenched and limbs flailed.

A nurse wheeled the sick man into the main area and quickly hooked up an oxygen mask, heart monitor leads and an intravenous line. Blood pressure: sixty over thirty, dangerously low. Heart rate: thirty five, also too low. The man suffered a seizure because not enough blood and oxygen could get to his brain due to a slow heartbeat. Some intravenous medication and fluids sent his vital signs back to normal range. He had, in fact, suffered a heart attack which showed itself in a deceptive way – causing pain primarily in his left shoulder joint area. His screening process did little to drill deeper into why a relatively young man had shoulder pain without any apparent injury. Another key error: his secondary symptom of dizziness that he never mentioned nor was asked about.

Triage is notoriously flawed and dependent upon the clinical experience and competence of the triage nurse. Overcrowding causes triage staff to rush still faster, leading to omissions in getting needed history or spotting the subtly sick folks. Older adults also develop more subtle and less typical manifestations of diseases, as mentioned, placing them at greater risk during the initial evaluation or triage process.

Most triage systems include a few major ingredients that will determine your priority to be seen:

- **Chief complaint** (most important): This factor is notoriously inaccurate because all people have different symptoms and presentations of illness that deviate from textbook descriptions. Folks also perceive and describe what they feel in quite different ways. Personal descriptions may vary depending upon individual pain tolerance, language barriers, education level or whether self-treatment with medication preceded the ER visit. Moreover, with older folks you might as well throw out the textbooks; they are particularly prone to showing *less typical* signs and symptoms of an illness. Older folks also may have difficulty describing symptoms in detail due to confusion from acute illness or medication, memory loss, or hearing or speech deficits. It is not unusual, for example, to have a chief complaint of "back pain" when experiencing a serious heart or lung problem. Moderate back pain would likely get a middling to low urgency ranking from triage systems. Disease can be deadly deceptive.

- **Appearance** is another factor triage nurses (or doctors) must consider as a priority, and has nothing to do with Prada purses or Sergio Rossi shoes. Once again, appearances can be quite deceptive. A stoic, retired laborer might seem okay on the outside when disease is boiling over inside. Inexperienced triage nurses or doctors, during a hurried assessment without much privacy, might overlook subtle clues of serious illness such as chest muscle contractions caused by breathing compromise, profuse sweating, pale face, or mottled coloring to arms or legs.
- **Vital signs:** These, too, can be misleading with older age. Older folks frequently do not spike fevers. Furthermore, seniors might, for instance, have a normally high blood pressure of 154 systolic. When the triage nurse measures a pressure of 110 systolic —lower than usual because of serious infection or dehydration— that would be considered "normal" and "stable" in triage software programs. Nurses would also file away in their minds that vital signs are "stable." Heart rate might be *falsely* normal, and not elevated, because of commonly used medications or heart scarring due to aging. Labored breathing is usually identifiable although older folks may have baseline respiratory ailments, thus obscuring worse air hunger. Sometimes, rapid or labored breathing is mistakenly labeled "anxiety." The anxiety is caused *by* the air hunger. If

someone wraps duct tape around your nose and mouth, you will quickly get anxious and panicky.

- **Pain level:** Older adults are more likely to have reduced pain perception, difficulty communicating details, and a tendency to understate symptoms so they don't "cause a fuss."
- **Acute versus chronic/recurring:** *Sudden* pain gets a step up in priority, *chronic* pain (or other symptoms) gets bumped down in priority. But some stoic folks have a high pain level and hide it well, while others moan and wince from the slightest discomfort. This deceptive disconnect between actual pain severity and the extent to which somebody moans, yells, gesticulates and grimaces can prove to be deadly. For chronic pain or other long-present symptoms, you are likely to be tossed into a low-urgency pile, leading to an extended wait. Even worse, you may see a lot of eye-rolling and will not be taken seriously for going to an ER for a chronic problem. Perhaps an urgent care or family doctor visit would be wiser? The exception: If that chronic problem suddenly got much more severe than usual on that day you seek care.
- **Past medical history** of chronic diseases can signal concern to triage nurses. Tell the screener your two or three major chronic ailments that could be relevant to your current problem. Caveat: There will not be time to go through elaborate medical histories. Save the full biography for the doctor who evaluates you. On the other hand, "I think this back pain is similar to what I had when I suffered a heart attack five years ago" is relevant past history for your triage spiel. Bring with you the name and contact information of your family doctor so emergency room staff can get any essential details or update your status.

Your Triage Spiel: A Matter of Life and Death

- Mention your chief complaint, but pay close attention to less prominent *secondary symptoms* that may signal serious illness. Examples include fever, extreme weakness, air hunger or breathing heaviness, dizziness, or feeling faint. Also watch for signs that accompany ominous organ-based (visceral) pain such as nausea, profuse sweating, restlessness or anxiety, or feelings of impending doom.

- Avoid mentioning every ache or pain you have experienced the past few weeks. It distracts from your chief complaint and wastes precious triage time. Your triage spiel must be short and sweet. Save those details for the doctor, if asked. On the other hand, if you are the stoic and gritty type who wrestles bears and alligators for fun, by all means tell the nurse and doctor this crucial information. If your pain now brings you to tears, this info will give you more street 'cred' that your sickness is potentially serious.
- Think about specific patterns of your major ailment. Is it worst ever? A problem you recognize from the past? Severe and constant from the outset? On and off the past few hours to days? Does anything seem to make the problem better? Worse?
- Have you tried simple remedies for the major complaint such as over-the-counter medications or prescriptions? Non-drug therapies? Any success? Did you get evaluated by another doctor? Have any tests been performed during the past few days? Started any new medications or supplements? Were you at another emergency room recently for the same problem? Multiple ER visits should serve as a red flag that serious illness might be simmering. Having tried failed remedies or gone through recent medical visits for the same concern adds credibility to your triage spiel.
- Bring a legible and updated list of your current medications and doses, or a sack filled with drug bottles if you are not yet organized. Do not forget off-the-shelf remedies, creams, eye drops, refrigerated or injectable medications, and herbals or supplements.
- Know your medication allergies, if any.

Triage time is up. Will you now receive quality or sub-par care? Keep alert or have an advocate with you. Ask questions. Do not be shy or timid. Call out for help if needed. Be polite. Know who is treating you. You are well on your way to healing.

Additional Triage Tips that may Save Your Life

1. Ask the nurse what your assigned triage level is and a ballpark estimate of the waiting time. For less serious illness, it can help you decide if urgent care, a family doctor appointment, or a free-standing emergency room might be a better option. Triage levels 4 and 5 are lowest priority and might require a long wait during busy times.

2. Emergency room workers are required to reassess folks waiting out in the waiting area, especially if they are deteriorating. But do not count on that. You must take the initiative and declare that you feel quite ill and need immediate attention. Explain politely that you need to rest on a stretcher. No time for etiquette if the ER staff dismisses your concerns. Your life depends upon it! Paradoxically, patients may feel too sick to get up and walk back to triage. This is a red flag that something is amiss. Ask anybody for assistance immediately to get back to triage or have an advocate go to bat for you.

3. It is highly advisable to bring an advocate with you when seeking emergency care. You will not be able to pay attention to detail while feeling sick. Your spouse, relative or friend can keep a list of any tests performed to avoid billing surprises, help with details of when you fell ill, and keep on top of ER staff regarding your medical care, testing, pain management, and basic needs such as a urinal or glass of water.

4. Keep cool. Do not scream and flail hysterically if not evaluated immediately. Politely ask the triage nurse for a reevaluation if deteriorating health-wise. If the nurse will not take your request seriously, ask to speak with a doctor. If that request hits a wall, call the hospital's patient advocate to get some concrete help. The exception: you might, as a last resort, be forced to moan and flail and do snow angels on the waiting room floor if all else fails. Staff will be forced to bring you into the emergency department on a stretcher. Your life might depend upon quicker evaluation if feeling seriously ill. The cleaning bill for your clothes dirtied on the floor, however, will be your responsibility.

5. Tell the triage nurse if you have had a recent hospitalization, rehab or nursing home stay since your current illness could be a direct result of procedures done or contact with dangerous hospital-based infections.
6. For those with a history of heart disease, it is wise to keep a miniaturized laminated copy of your electrocardiogram in your purse or wallet. For tech savvy folks, have the file available on your smartphone. Doctors will want to compare the new EKG with the old one to search for any changes in zigzag patterns.
7. You or your advocate might want to ask the triage nurse which provider will be evaluating you. Will it be an emergency care physician? A doctor who is moonlighting or filling in a weekend shift to earn extra cash (but is completing training in an unrelated specialty)? A nurse practitioner or physician assistant? A young medical student or doctor in training? It is important to know the training and experience of the person wearing the scrubs or white coat. If you have any doubts about your condition, are not improving, or do not have faith in the provider caring for you, you have the right to request that an ER physician in charge or specialist offer another opinion.
8. The triage nurse might order some tests to expedite your evaluation. Triage is the one place where you can let it ride and allow a simple x-ray or blood test to be ordered without a doctor explaining risks versus benefits. Those tests will likely make logical sense like basic screening blood tests for food poisoning or an ankle x-ray for an obvious injury.

DANGER 3. MEDICATION MADNESS: DRUG OVERUSE IN OLDER ADULTS

"I firmly believe that if the whole materia medica (medications), as now used, could be sunk to the bottom of the sea, it would be all the better for mankind— and all the worse for the fishes."

Oliver Wendell Holmes, noted American physician and author

"To write a prescription is easy, but to come to an understanding with people is hard."

Author Franz Kafka, in "A Country Doctor"

Medications can heal and medications can harm. Finding balance is essential since no drug is completely safe. What is more concerning is that older adults are at greatest risk. Medical experts have for decades discussed how preventable bad reactions to medications can be; yet, the problem remains a growing concern today for adults and the elderly. It seems that older folks are prescribed more and more "must-have" medications to treat more and more "must-treat" chronic illnesses. As we age, the balance scale tips toward the side of harm from taking medications for several reasons:

- As we grow older, our kidneys work less efficiently at processing toxins in our system.
- The aging liver is no longer as competent at neutralizing toxins and chemicals.
- Our muscle mass melts into fat with each passing decade. The result: the effects drugs have on our body persist longer and may reach toxic levels.
- Other chronic diseases can be made worse by medication side effects. For instance, anti-inflammatory pain killers for arthritis can cause the blood pressure to soar, heart failure to worsen, and heart attack risk to increase slightly. Overactive bladder drugs can

cause confusion and behavior changes in those with and without baseline memory loss.

- Many doctors use the same medication doses for a 40-year old and a 70-year old adult without considering drug processing ability as mentioned above.
- With each medication added to an older adult's list, chances for drug reactions skyrocket. These effects are additive and can include vague deterioration such as loss of appetite and weight, general functional decline, fatigue, falls and memory difficulties.

Consider the following examples of potential consequences from prescribing run amuck:

It seemed like grandma's time was up. After nine decades, her sharp mind had dulled from dementia, her lungs were ravaged by asthma, her heart was damaged from high blood pressure and blocked arteries, and now her kidneys failed fast. The long medication list she was expected to take resembled a list of ingredients for a complicated dinner recipe. While on the subject of recipes, not even the tastiest of them could spark her now diminished appetite. She had recently lost eighteen pounds. Grandma was given sedatives and sleeping pills for anxiety and behavioral issues due to dementia; heart and high blood pressure pills; memory loss pills; as well as antidepressants, blood thinners, stomach acid-lowering and asthma drugs. Thirteen different drugs in total! It seemed crystal clear she was at the end of her hospice rope, growing increasingly confused, agitated, restless. Her new hospice doctor then had a Eureka moment. The doctor stopped many of her medications which could have affected her mind, kidneys and body as a whole. Over the next two months, like a prayer answered, grandma's mind cleared up significantly, her appetite returned as she packed on the pounds, and she could walk again for short distances without falling! Her failing kidneys cleared the cobwebs and cranked back up to par. She could now speak in longer phrases and participate in group activities, greatly improving her quality of life. This apparent medical miracle, a true anecdote published in a 2014 edition of the journal *Annals of Long-term Care,* happened after her list of medications went from thirteen-long down to five. In fact, this "medical miracle" happens every day in nursing homes, assisted living facilities and care homes across the United States and the globe as more care providers realize the dangers of over-medication or polypharmacy.

*

A retired music industry writer had notched many chronic ailments under his 80-year old belt. He was diagnosed with dementia, bladder cancer, back pain after spine surgery, high blood pressure, diabetes, acid reflux, gastritis and chronic kidney disease from aging. This was not uncommon beyond the eighth decade and his list of over a dozen medications also struck a familiar note. Mr. S took blood thinners and other medications for his heart, memory loss, pain, diabetes, and high cholesterol. His life routine remained fixated on following his wife around the house and little else. He was forgetful and fell often. Quality of life was absent. When his doctor tapered him off of several drugs including gabapentin and etodolac for pain, digoxin for the heart, and iron supplements he made positive strides. He stopped falling and soon went to yoga classes with his wife and exercised at the gym regularly. This is a summary of an actual case report that appeared in an October 2010 issue of *Journal of the American Medical Association.*

*

Mrs. K seemed to be doing well lately. She was eating better and in good spirits despite her frail condition and recent hospitalization. This great grandmother had even been sitting outside a few minutes each day while the weather was nice. Her caregiver was shocked to find Mrs. K gasping for air a few days later. Mrs. K was rushed to the emergency room by ambulance and diagnosed with aspiration pneumonia. Her caregiver had no way of knowing that Mrs. K's medications, prescribed to enhance her medical condition, were actually multiplying her risks for aspiration. A few of the culprit drugs were: sleeping pill; potent pain pill; acid-lowering drug to "protect the stomach," yet it imperiled her lungs; and her overactive bladder medication. Many unrelated drugs all have in common cumulative risk for aspiration pneumonia.

Risk-Benefit Classification of Medications

I have compartmentalized medications into several tidy descriptive categories based upon the benefits versus risks of use.

New and Unproven Drugs

These are medications that should be avoided like the plague, unless it is a fight for life and no other drugs are available. When a drug gets approval for use, perhaps a few thousand people have taken the medication in clinical studies during the approval process. The true "guinea pig" phase is the millions of patients prescribed a newfangled medication *after* Food and Drug Administration (FDA) approval. Several thousand test subjects are not enough users to discover less common, more serious reactions to a drug. Vioxx, for instance, became a billion dollar pain drug before the reports of increased heart attack risk were taken seriously enough to pull that drug off the market. Dabigatran, a newfangled blood thinner, serves as another example of new and concerning medications.

Hidden and Hushed Dangers of Medication: Dabigatran

The concerning clues and hints of danger dribbled in but that did not stop the drug dabigatran from achieving blockbuster status. This new blood thinner, used to prevent strokes in people with an irregular heart rhythm called atrial fibrillation, was touted to cause fewer bleeding complications than warfarin (affectionately called rat poison by many patients). Dabigatran rocketed to drug stardom because, unlike warfarin, this "new and improved" blood thinner boasted no need for careful blood level monitoring. Without frequent blood testing, dabigatran liberated both patients and doctors. Or so it was thought by those who were prescribed this new medication.

Reports surfaced in 2011 about a spike in *fatal* bleeding episodes in those on this newfangled drug. Then there were murmurs about an increased risk for heart attack in the one major study on which the FDA based approval of the drug. Furthermore, as Deborah Cohen, Investigations Editor for the *British Medical Journal*, reports in a July 2014 issue of that publication, the 'RE-LY' trial had significant flaws. The FDA usually requires two major studies for drug approval but dabigatran scooted by with only one big study. In addition, many important study patient events were omitted then later found during the approval process, causing some experts to have concerns about the validity of the study. It later came to light that the manufacturer knew serious bleeding complications could be reduced by up to 40 percent if blood levels of the drug were monitored and adjusted—just like with warfarin. But hold on! The crucial selling point of this star medication was *not* needing blood monitoring. Who stood to suffer most from this disturbing safety concern? The elderly. Older folks are more susceptible to serious bleeding complications as are people who have kidney disease. Sadly, newly developed medications are sometimes developed and approved under murky circumstances.

Useless Drugs

Useless medications are those with few actual benefits for people taking the drug. Ezetimibe, a cholesterol-lowering drug, was found in a major study called ENHANCE to reduce cholesterol levels but had no benefit on actual plaque buildup within neck arteries. Why lower cholesterol levels if that doesn't lead to actual reduced risk for heart attack or stroke? The IMPROVE-IT trial result recently found some health benefits when ezetimibe was added to a statin drug to lower cholesterol immediately following a heart attack. Despite this very limited benefit in a specific heart attack population, many doctors in the United States and Canada continue to prescribe the drug routinely to simply lower cholesterol numbers in people without any history of heart attack. The benefits from taking this drug just to lower cholesterol are dubious at best. In fact, the American Heart Association's most recent guidelines have de-emphasized the importance of focusing on a specific cholesterol number. Many drugs are used nowadays to lower a high number such as cholesterol or blood pressure without any studies proving the medication leads to fewer bad events or longer survival.

Iffy Benefits and Many Risks

Memory drugs such as donepezil and memantine may be poster children for the iffy benefits and many risks category. These drugs are prescribed as magic pills in nursing homes and assisted living facilities across the globe. The reason: Hope. No other treatments are available for this devastating disease called Alzheimer's. Another reason: Excellent marketing by drug companies. Yet a 2008 *Annals of Internal Medicine* review of all studies done testing these memory drugs concluded that these medications had marginal benefits for dementia. A few of the deficiencies in the evidence included:

- Most studies lasted less than one year
- Most study subjects were fairly healthy other than dementia; real-world dementia sufferers are often frail and have many other chronic ailments that predispose them to bad drug reactions.
- The studies did not pay much attention to quality of life, function and behavioral effects of taking the drugs – the most important measures of benefit for caregivers and patients.
- Statistically significant benefit in these studies, for example, was a 3-point higher test score of general thinking function on a 70-item test. This minimal improvement is hardly a result worth suffering many potential side effects for.
- Real-world side effect reports appear to be far more common and severe than those reported in these studies of fairly healthy folks. Just to name a few: loss of appetite, stomach upset, vomiting, diarrhea, weakness, irritability, restlessness, delusions, blood pressure abnormalities, heart arrhythmias. A new Veterans Affairs health system study, in fact, has shown these dementia drugs are associated with significant weight loss in many older folks.

Perhaps the significant money spent on these drugs would be better invested in more caregiver help and emphasis on creative engagement and quality of life. It has been estimated that dementia sufferers receive caregiver interaction only about two hours out of each 24-hour day. In fact, these drugs might become an excuse for caregivers not to engage with these folks as much since "They are already being treated with medication for the memory problem."

A second example of iffy benefits but plenty of risk is use of cholesterol-lowering drugs called 'statins' (lovastatin, pravastatin, simvastatin, atorvastatin, rosuvastatin) by adults who have *not* ever suffered a heart attack or stroke. The evidence from studies shows about one person will be spared a heart attack for every 100 people who take the statin drug everyday for five years. However, many of these people will suffer daily side effects that reduce quality of life such as muscle pains, weakness, diabetes, stomach ailments, and possibly brain fog. The drug labeling for statin drugs must now include a warning about the risk for developing diabetes (2% incidence overall, but up to 9% diabetes risk in older adults) and memory loss from taking these drugs. This drug warning requirement was finally implemented in 2012. In fact, there is evidence that older adults with the lowest levels of cholesterol have higher death rates! Exercise and proper diet are treatments that have no serious side effects and benefits can be as good as, or better than, drug treatments.

For elderly folks with a known history of heart attack or stroke, 'statin' drugs can be beneficial if the side effects are tolerable. This decision must be made based upon each person's risk-benefit assessment.

It is important to note that 'statin' drugs block an enzyme that leads to production of cholesterol; however, production of many other important proteins and hormones can also be blocked as a result. For instance, Coenzyme Q10, sex hormones, steroid hormones, vitamin D and other enzyme proteins needed for key body functions may be blocked by statin drugs. There is good evidence that 'statin' drugs cause damage to cell mitochondria, the energy production factory of cells. Brain and muscle cells need to quickly boost energy supplies to accommodate life functions, but may not get sufficient energy when 'statin' drugs block these vital chemicals and proteins. This could explain the muscle pain, fatigue and brain fog side effects attributed to these medications, according to the research of Dr. Beatrice Golomb, an expert on adverse drug effects. Who is most at risk of suffering these negative effects? Why, of course, it is older folks.

Good Benefits and Low Risks

There are many medications that offer better health and quality of life yet have few significant side effects. A few examples include allergy medications like loratadine, albuterol for asthma, and acetaminophen for mild to moderate pain. When the choice for a senior is to suffer all day from neck pain or to take acetaminophen to dull the pain, it is an easy decision. Acetaminophen is safe in doses under 3000 mg per day. Exceptions: those who abuse alcohol or suffer from serious liver disease.

Good Benefits Versus High Risks

The blood thinner warfarin is an example of a drug that can prevent a stroke in those with atrial fibrillation, but can also cause life-threatening bleeding. Frequent blood level monitoring and dietary restrictions while taking warfarin can diminish quality of life as well.

Unforeseen Consequences of Medication Use

Side effects, known as adverse drug effects, are usually readily apparent negative consequences of taking medication. But it doesn't end there. Many unexpected and less obvious consequences of medication use exist as well.

1. Medication use can lead to **unintended consequences** even if properly prescribed. For instance, taking 'statin' drugs to lower cholesterol had an odd effect in older men, according to a 2014 study printed in *Journal of the American Medical Association Internal Medicine*. While these men took the cholesterol drugs, they showed a significant drop in exercise levels and seemed more sedentary overall. Possible explanations: A side effect of the medication is muscle pain or fatigue. Another reason could be that the study subjects felt there is no need for exercise since the drug will do all the hard work. That is a common danger of taking any medication – developing a sense of external locus of control, meaning these people might depend only on outside help to improve health rather than using self-motivation and inner empowerment techniques.

2. **Serious, subtle, side effects**: Suffering from a rash is easy to identify, but oftentimes serious yet subtle side effects occur when taking medication. These effects can be difficult to identify. For example, there are many reports by people taking 'statin' drugs that they experience a brain fogginess and memory issues. As another example, a recent study reaffirmed the concern that popping anticholinergic drugs – which include old antihistamines like diphenhydramine, overactive bladder drugs, and some less common medications like amitriptyline – is linked to *long-term* memory decline. Clearly, subtle and not-so-subtle adverse medication effects can

reduce quality of life by causing fatigue or muscle pain or weakness, confusion and other negative effects.

3. **'LazyRx' use**: In the typical rush and chaos of medical practice, doctors commonly use what I call the 'LazyRx' technique. By writing a prescription for treatment, medical care providers have an excuse for quickly ending the visit without more detailed communication, explanation and history taking. This lazy technique also serves as substitute for equally important guidance on lifestyle modifications which require much discussion time.
4. Many drugs have minimal to modest benefits at best but are often prescribed for **lack of any better treatment**. Even effective drugs might not be beneficial in frail elderly folks since research studies usually exclude the frail elder population. In frail folks, side effects might outweigh any benefits. Long-term benefits may not have sufficient time to materialize in the very old who have limited life expectancy.
5. Other problems with medication include **drug-drug interactions** that are unexpected or additive, as well as drugs that make other *diseases* worse (**drug-disease interaction**). Taking ibuprofen for arthritis pain, for instance, can lead to higher blood pressure levels. Alternatively, a medication can cause a 'new' disease; for instance, some beta blockers for heart ailments can cause depression symptoms. Some doctors might then prescribe an antidepressant drug for this 'new' problem rather than simply removing the first culprit medication. This is called "**cascade prescribing**."
6. **"Lifer-Drugs"**: Once a drug is prescribed, future doctors may be reluctant to ever remove that medication or lower the dosage out of misguided fear the patient might suffer a terrible health insult and blame that newer doctor.
7. If you are given antibiotics for a viral illness **what harm can it do** to take the drug a few days? This common scenario can create, in essence, a Frankenstein laboratory within you that is giving life to brawny bacteria that are now resistant to common antibiotics. In addition, if you suffer significant antibiotic side effects like

vomiting or diarrhea you will wish you simply rode out the virus with fluids and bed rest.

8. **Kidney Crash**: As we age our kidneys work less efficiently so we are unable to process these medications as well as a younger adult. The result can be high levels of that drug within the body causing serious side effects or wreaking havoc on the kidneys. All people over age 40 should get a basic blood test to find out their blood 'creatinine' level. That value can be entered into www.mdrd.com entry fields along with age, sex and race. Check the box near 'Chronic kidney disease (GFR less than 60)'… and voila! You can get your "**K-Stage**," as I call it. K-stage is your stage of chronic kidney disease, if present. Chronic kidney damage can be present despite a "normal" range creatinine value on a blood test. When a small, elderly woman has a high-normal creatinine level, that might reflect significant kidney disease since an elderly woman has far less muscle mass than the general population. Creatinine is a breakdown product of muscle. With less muscle mass, a thin lady should have a very low blood creatinine value. A 'high normal' creatinine level in the elderly often represents actual chronic kidney disease. Less lean muscle mass translates into reduced ability to metabolize medications.
9. **Over-the-counter medications** can also cause serious side effects. Ibuprofen and aspirin taken for long periods of time can cause kidney damage, raise blood pressure or carve out stomach ulcers. Seemingly innocuous ranitidine or famotidine to lower stomach acid can cause confusion, hallucinations and delirium. Seniors are at greatest risk for these adverse reactions that can be quite shocking when we think of off-the-shelf drugs as being harmless.
10. **Medication Confusion**: With each additional pill to pop, chances rise that mistakes will be made in taking that complex drug regimen. Errors in dosing or overdosing can land folks in the hospital.
11. **Gray-haired Guinea Pigs**: As mentioned earlier, most drug studies include a small number of subjects, perhaps a few thousand, who are tested for benefits and dangers over a short period of time such as one to three years. What's more, these test subjects are primarily

younger and healthier adults. Few are elderly and rarely will frail, old folks be tested in studies. So when grandma takes a medication for her ailment, the sixth drug on her list, she is essentially a guinea pig. She has become a test subject for effects of that drug on seniors who have many ailments and who take many medications. Side effects can cause serious complications in the elderly such as falls or loss of appetite, for instance. Researchers seeking drug approval could never study these complex, frail folks in testing a drug for risk versus benefit. The drug would likely never get approval due to too many adverse reactions and complicating factors in a sicker population. What's more, adults who get prescriptions for these medications are expected to take these medications for many years or a lifetime! Study subjects usually are tested for a year or two maximum. Nobody yet knows a new drug's long-term safety.

12. **Under Five, Stay Alive**: The risk for an adverse drug reaction in older folks is 13 percent when taking two drugs. That bad reaction risk soars to 82 percent when taking seven or more medications! In other words, as more drugs of any kind are added to the daily medication list, the risk for negative effects skyrockets. At least 100,000 older adults are *hospitalized* each year in the United States because of adverse reactions to prescribed or off- the-shelf medications. Many more folks are treated and released from emergency rooms across the country after suffering an adverse drug event. Take only essential drugs and keep the list short – under five, if possible – to limit drug interactions and reactions.

Power of Positive and Negative Thinking

Why bother trying non-drug approaches to ailments such as exercise, proper diet, meditation, music, yoga, martial arts, acupuncture, engagement in creative activities, herbal remedies and many others? Both positive and negative thinking cause release of brain chemicals that parallel the effects many medications have on our brain and body, according to recent research. The simple therapeutic acts of caring, compassion and touching cause release of many active body chemicals that are similarly released by the actions of drugs. What's more, words are perhaps the most powerful tool in the doctor's bag. Studies have found that when doctors tell patients a new drug they will take can cause vomiting and diarrhea, for instance, more people who were told this actually experienced those side effects even though they were given a harmless sugar pill.

In a well received Harvard study, Dr. Ted Kaptchuk divided 262 people who suffered from irritable bowel syndrome into three groups: No treatment; fake or sham acupuncture without much said by the care provider; and fake acupuncture done with 20 minutes of exaggerated compassion, touch and caring by the provider. Needless to say, those in the third group experienced the greatest relief of symptoms despite getting fake treatment.

Dr. Kaptchuk then took it one step further and told participants in another study they were getting a placebo (sugar pill) treatment. The control group was told they were getting no treatment. Irritable bowel syndrome sufferers who were told they would get a placebo (sugar pill) as treatment experienced twice as much symptom relief as those told they would not get any treatment! In fact, it has been shown that people who expect to die going into surgery are more likely to have delayed recovery and serious complications. Non-verbal clues telegraphed by doctors or nurses to seriously ill patients can also have significant effects on those people. Clearly, belief and effort in trying *non-drug* therapies can have very real and positive effects on mind and body. This is particularly true for exercise and healthful eating. These nondrug approaches are surely worth a try and guess what? No negative side effects. With health and medical treatments, sometimes believing is seeing.

Sobering Stats and Facts

The following eye-opening facts and stats serve as reminder that there may be a steep price to pay when taking any medication. A careful assessment of risks and benefits is crucial using your own research as well as your doctor's explanation. First-line treatment, of course, should always be lifestyle changes or simple and safe nondrug therapies. Remember the power of positive thinking in the placebo effect.

- About one in every 20 unplanned hospitalizations is medication related and adverse drug reactions are responsible for about 10 percent of hospital admissions in older folks.

- Those who take sleep aid medications have a death rate three to five times higher than nonusers, according to a large study published in the *British Medical Journal Open* 2012. An increased cancer link was also found. Drugs considered hypnotics for sleep include zolpidem and similar 'Z-drugs', temazepam, diazepam, barbiturates, and sedating antihistamines such as diphenhydramine. Warm milk, hot bath and daytime exercise are looking quite appealing as insomnia remedies right about now.
- Older folks are about seven times more likely to be hospitalized for a bad reaction to medication than are younger adults.
- A 2011 *New England Journal of Medicine* study found four common classes of drugs to be responsible for the majority of serious adverse drug events leading to emergency room visits or hospitalization. Many more bad reactions remain unreported or unrecognized as a drug side effect by both doctors and patients. The four drug types are insulins; warfarin (blood thinner); platelet inhibitors (type of blood thinner); and pills used for diabetic blood sugar control. Other studies identified digoxin as another trouble-maker drug for older adults. Each person must weigh risks and benefits of taking these riskier drugs. For instance, some major studies that compare aspirin versus warfarin for stroke prevention showed that warfarin bested aspirin by only one percent (1.4% strokes per year versus 2.39% for aspirin). However, other studies found warfarin to cause significantly more serious bleeding episodes. This number can easily go higher in the real world where oversight is more lax than in a study setting. The question older folks at risk for stroke must ask: Is this small decrease in stroke risk worth the frequent blood tests and higher bleeding dangers? Not a simple answer. Regarding diabetes medications, frail seniors must consider if they really will benefit from overly tight blood sugar control which can lead to hypoglycemia (low sugar) hospitalizations.
- A recent study found that many people believe that drugs approved by the Food and Drug Administration are uniformly effective and safe from serious side effects. In fact, many drugs have only marginal actual benefits and most serious side effects come to light

after millions of prescriptions are written when the drug is already approved for marketing and sale to the public!

- The European Medicines Agency recently recommended halting sale of nearly fifty drugs, according to a Medscape.com news alert, due to concerns about drug testing integrity and methods used by GVK Biosciences, a pharmaceutical contract research organization in Hyderabad, India. Flawed clinical studies mostly for generic equivalents conducted by this research company underlie the decision, according to Medscape.com. Clearly, just because a drug is for sale and is being prescribed, does not mean it is truly safe and effective.
- A 2007 report from the Institute of Medicine estimated that between 380,000 and 450,000 preventable adverse drug events occurred annually in United States hospitals.
- Adverse drug events cause over 700,000 emergency department visits each year in the United States. Nearly 120,000 patients each year need to be hospitalized for further treatment after emergency visits for these bad reactions.
- Between six and 30 percent of people who are hospitalized experience a negative medication reaction during their hospitalization.
- Adverse drug events are quite common after hospitalizations because many medication changes can lead to mix-ups.
- Many specialists prescribe the latest, newest drug or risky treatment since they are the last hope for folks who might have failed simpler remedies. Reputation is also enhanced when a specialist offers the latest fashions in therapy. Bear in mind, however, that a specialist is more likely to do tests and procedures and prescribe medications to address your ailments.
- Avoid falling victim to prescribing fads. For instance, stomach acid-lowering medications (PPIs, H2 blockers) are overprescribed across the globe. Some studies found that as many as 70 percent of hospitalized adults receive these medications without an appropriate reason and contrary to accepted guidelines. While many doctors believe hospitalized patients benefit from stress ulcer-preventing

drugs, these folks end up taking these medications indefinitely after discharge home. The problem: we need acid in our stomachs! It kills invading bacteria to reduce infection risk. The acidity is also necessary for proper absorption of many essential nutrients like vitamin B12, iron, magnesium and calcium. The most-feared theoretical effect of long-term use of these drugs include overgrowth of special cells in the stomach as they try to compensate for lack of an acid environment. These enterochromaffin-like cells can possibly transform into aggressive cancerous cells.

Tips to Remember

1. Drug dosages used are commonly too high for aging folks who have less muscle mass, reduced kidney function and take many other medications. 'Start low and go slow' is the golden rule when medications are necessary for seniors.
2. Never put medications in bottles that are improperly labeled.
3. Store essential medications in a cool and dry place, rendering the humid bathroom medicine chest less than ideal.
4. If an older adult experiences any new symptom, it should be considered an adverse side effect or reaction to a medication, unless proven otherwise.
5. Older folks, especially those in the latter years of their lives, are faced with prescriptions for medication that perhaps may offer a slight and theoretical benefit to extend life, but could crush quality of life. Each individual must decide what is right for them.
6. Expect full **informed consent** from the prescriber for a new medication just as you would for a surgical procedure. Use the IC Q-kits described in the Informed Consent chapter of this book. "Take this pill, it will make you feel better" is simply not good enough. Ask hardball questions: How long has the medication been around? Is it safe? How effective will it be for my ailment? Have studies shown it has clear benefits or are benefits only marginal? What are the most common and most severe side effects? Can this drug make my other chronic diseases worse or interact

with other medication I am taking? What can we try first that does not involve taking a drug? Here is another key concept to discuss with your provider about taking a medication: Do drug approval studies show actual health benefits like lower risk for heart attack, for instance? Or do the studies only show a secondary or indirect benefit like lowering cholesterol numbers without proof stroke and heart attack risk drops too? Do your own research as well. Are published critiques of the major studies scathing? Do analyses of drug approval studies question their conclusions as unconvincing because of flaws in the methods used? Have there been journal articles published about concerning patterns of serious side effects? Recall that medication safety and effectiveness in a study are usually modest even under ideal study conditions, in a relatively healthy and carefully selected group of study participants! That is nothing like the real world effects the medication might have.

7. Drugs must never be first choice treatment unless the illness is immediately life-threatening. Try improving diet, exercising, gardening, reducing stress, yoga, Tai Chi, meditation, acupuncture, physical therapy and other nondrug remedies before agreeing to take a medication.

8. Direct-to-consumer ads may propagate the perception that people always want a drug treatment when they ask for more information about these drugs. Doctors then feel pressured to prescribe medication whether or not it is truly the best option. Be careful of what you ask from your doctor, or you may get it!

9. Beware the "RxFlex!" This is my label for a reflexive response that commonly afflicts healthcare providers. The mere mention of a symptom or ailment is followed quickly by whipping out the prescription pad, like a gunslinger drawing his gun. Insomnia serves as an example. When a patient complains of difficulty sleeping many providers reflexively suggest and then immediately write an Rx for a sleep aid. Yet, they have barely asked for details about why the person cannot sleep. Simple solutions may be effective like avoiding caffeinated drinks at night, increasing daytime exercise, avoiding daytime naps, learning coping strategies for stress,

calming music, warm baths, and treatment of medical conditions that directly contribute to insomnia. Many medications can also affect sleep quality. If your doctor reaches for his Rx pad before asking detailed questions about your ailment, run, run, run. Or simply exert your Patient Power and say, "No! Thanks."

10. Never allow someone to give you a medication in the hospital or nursing home, especially intravenously, unless they confirm *you* should be getting it and explain what the drug is, the dosage, and why you are receiving it.
11. Specialists tend to prescribe more medications including the newest contenders. This might be a good thing for someone who is very sick and other treatments have failed to help. For the usual chronic ailments, older folks must be cautious about seeking specialist care for less serious problems. The specialist will likely end up ordering more tests and prescribing more drugs or higher doses of established medications.
12. Some additional key considerations with medications: Are there any dietary restrictions like when taking warfarin? The timing for taking a drug can be significant as well. It is not uncommon for older folks to be taking three drugs that lower blood pressure – all given in the morning. Blood pressure control should be spread out over 24 hours. Furthermore, those three drugs can bottom out grandma's pressure if taken all at once, leading to fainting or a broken hip. Does a medication cause drowsiness or weakness? Perhaps that drug should be taken at bedtime.
13. If you agree to take a medication for valid reasons, ask if a cheaper generic drug would be similarly effective at treating your problem. That generic drug can save you a lot of money, get the same results, and might be safer since it has been around for many years, unlike the untested new kid on the block.

Top 10 Reasons Doctors Prescribe Medications to People:

1. "Patients want the doctor to take action when they are sick so they will get some action," the doctor says to himself. Go to the pharmacy. Fill the prescription. Pay big bucks. Swallow a bitter pill. Get side effects. Feel better???

2. Drug sales reps tell doctors about the many wonders of the medications they promote. Doctors like to please sales reps. If they write many prescriptions then they might be offered speaker status and do talks on the "benefits" of the drug and earn easy money. They then may get to travel to warm, sunny destinations with all expenses paid.

3. Drug samples are a great way to get patients out the door quickly. Folks like getting free stuff. It keeps them distracted from asking too many questions.

4. Many doctors believe it is always better to treat than not to. Years of doctor training focuses on actions they must take to make patients feel better—prescribing drugs, ordering tests, performing procedures. The days of hand-holding, communication, explanation, coaching and reassurance that most things get better on their own went out of vogue with the leeches.

5. Fear. Doctors fear patients will stare at them suspiciously and with enmity if they tell a patient there isn't much they can do for that problem. To add salt to the wound, the *patient* must do the hard work like tough it out a few days, or exercise and eat better and change bad habits or avoid vices. "I had to pay the doctor $150 for this?!!?!!"

6. Dread. If the patient gets worse, that person will conclude the doctor has a fake diploma and will never return for care. Negative word of mouth or online reviews could cost a lot of business for a principled doctor who does not give out useless prescriptions or perform avoidable or harmful procedures. Should patients always get the treatments they expect and ask for? Isn't medical care now based upon teamwork and mutual discussion between doctor and

patient? Hmmm… Be careful of what you ask for, or you may get it!

7. Sheer terror! What if no prescribed treatment leads to a possible bad outcome, or the disease just gets worse? Will a summons for malpractice litigation arrive at the doctor's doorstep? Simple but scary.
8. Hope. Maybe, just maybe, that prescription will actually nail it and make the patient feel better quickly. Maybe results are from the placebo effect? No matter. Happy patient equals more future visits which equals successful, smiley doctor. Glowing internet reviews and stellar reputation are priceless. Simple formula, really.
9. Clinical guidelines say so. For example: high cholesterol needs lowering. If a doctor does not prescribe a drug it can be considered 'sub-standard' care. Spending one hour explaining principles of nutrition and exercise is out of the question. Too much time wasted. Besides, the doctor's knowledge in that department might be a bit murky. Rx is all that is left to offer, if the provider can get the prescription written in the remaining one minute and forty-eight seconds of the visit. What is worse, sometimes these guidelines that doctors must follow are not aligned with an individual patient's wishes for care. Did the doctor ask what is most important to *you*, the patient?
10. Cool, newfangled drug. Might be worth a try on the next few guinea pigs that stroll through the office door. Will it work? Will it nearly kill the patient? Stay tuned…

DANGER 4. TEST WORSHIP: TOO MUCH TRUST IN TESTS

"Diagnostic certainty usually is unattainable; it is frequently not required for optimal care… the attempt to reach certainty with more and more tests sometimes produces substantial harm…"

Jerome P. Kassirer, MD
Former Editor, New England Journal of Medicine

"A laboratory test by itself rarely, if ever, establishes a clinical diagnosis."

Joseph S. Alpert, MD
Director of Coronary Care, University of Arizona College of Medicine
Editor-in-Chief, American Journal of Medicine

The elderly woman's low back MRI looked horrible, even to the radiologist. Narrowing of the spine canal. Arthritis changes throughout the bones in the spine (vertebrae). A herniated disc in the lower back. But the woman wasn't worried. Neither was the radiologist. How odd? Not really, because the woman had no back pain, was fully mobile and active. That is right - no pain, despite all those "abnormalities" on the MRI.

Several studies published during the earlier days of high-tech imaging discovered that doing an MRI or CT scan on folks who had no back symptoms at all often revealed many structural abnormalities in the spine. Finding these "abnormalities" of unclear importance on imaging is not without risks. A correlation has been identified between knowing one has test abnormalities and lower self-rating of health. It is termed *disease labeling*. Back pain sufferers who undergo MRI testing, for example, display more illness behavior and require more doctor visits than similar people who did not get imaging done. What's more concerning, researchers found that in parts of the United States where more MRIs are ordered for back pain, back surgery rates are higher too. Clearly, undergoing avoidable tests can have serious and risky consequences.

H. Michael Heuser, a Los Angeles film producer, was very worried about the perfusion CT scans he underwent at the Prestigious Cedars Sinai Medical Center in 2009, when he experienced stroke symptoms. Was he worried about the stroke? Sure, but he recovered from that. Soon after undergoing three special CT scans, he lost large clumps of hair and broke out with burning welts all over his body. He will surely fret over this for the rest of his life. An investigation discovered that he was exposed to **eight times** the usual radiation dose in error! The hair loss and rash – that was radiation poisoning! He may now have a lifetime cancer risk hundreds of times higher than the norm. According to media reports, hundreds of other folks were subjected to similar radiation poisoning during that time frame. The folly was presumed to be due to a combination of CT scan technologist errors and equipment software misuse.

Many people sanctify tests. Like primitive man's belief in magic as cause and cure for disease, modern-day patients mistakenly believe medical science and technology offer definite answers, quick cures. Patients might feel cheated and suspicious if a doctor does *not* order an x- ray or blood test – or something! We like high-tech. Smartphones are cool. Laptops increase our productivity. Tablets and e-readers are slick and convenient. Tests are reassuring – but is it *false* reassurance? Consider the elderly man who has a history of high blood pressure and suddenly develops dizziness. His brain CT scan at the emergency room is "negative," meaning no definite stroke is found. He is sent home, still dizzy, but reassured his motion sickness medication will help. What he has no way of knowing is that CT scan could miss up to 80 percent of strokes early on in people suffering from just the symptom of dizziness. A coin toss could have been more accurate!

You might be asking: "Why shouldn't I undergo the latest high-tech tests so I can have an accurate diagnosis and get better medical care?" Technology does often solve difficult diagnoses and thus can help doctors provide better care. The anecdote of the man with abdominal pain in Section III attests to that. This is true only when testing is done appropriately in those people most likely to have serious disease and who truly need imaging. Too often, however, imaging is performed indiscriminately and automatically, and sometimes with interests other than the best patient care. Excessive testing can lead to needless worry and unnecessary risky procedures. It is estimated that 1 in 7 emergency room patients age 65 and older receive a head CT scan! That's just the head. Other estimates suggest one-third of the 70 million CT scans done annually are not medically necessary. Ponder this: Far fewer tests are performed in Canada, adjusted for lower population, yet outcomes for illness and death rates are no worse.

Regarding the potential consequences of testing, consider the all-too-frequent problem of "incidentalomas" in hi-tech testing, which refers to unexpected test findings that could be normal body variation or an unimportant "abnormality." The case report of an elderly woman with persistent back pain who *appropriately* underwent an MRI of her spine serves as an eye-opening example. The spine imaging incidentally spotted a complex cyst in one of her kidneys which was not amenable to a needle biopsy. She ultimately underwent major surgery and had her kidney removed out of fear by doctors that it was cancer! Final diagnosis: harmless cyst that likely would never have affected her health.

In truth, tests provide doctors with clues and tidbits of information that they must interpret in context of who the patient is, what they are feeling, and their risk factors for having a serious ailment. Are you a test worshipper? Do you sanctify tests and believe it is always better to undergo testing, procedures and treatments to find an accurate diagnosis or achieve cure? Read on about the unreliability and inaccuracy of tests and it will surely turn your faith in tests into agnostic uncertainty.

Incorrect Diagnosis: All Too Common, Often Preventable

With all these tests being done, why do significant misdiagnoses occur up to 15 percent of the time in medical practice? Studies usually blame systems errors. Examples of system errors include established procedures for getting test results, automatically labeling a body part to be operated upon, or having best-practice checklists to follow when performing procedures. But quite often a diagnosis depends upon a single medical provider such as a doctor or nurse practitioner. That provider must formulate the correct list of diagnostic possibilities (differential diagnosis); order appropriate tests, if needed, beginning with simpler and safer options; have the necessary experience and expertise to measure up to this difficult task; know when to ask for help; and have that sixth sense of knowing when a patient is very sick and when more must be done regardless of what test results may suggest.

Following are a few reasons doctors and nurse practitioners commonly misdiagnose a patient's ailment even under the best of circumstances:

- **Inexperience or lack of proper expertise**: For instance, a gastroenterology Fellow (still in final training) works a weekend ER shift to earn extra money and treats heart attack victims; an intern (doctor-in-training) cares for you at a teaching hospital emergency room; or a newbie ER doctor or nurse practitioner fully manages your complex care without input from more experienced doctors.
- **Diagnostic Bias**: Those who diagnose disease usually develop a

working diagnosis within seconds based upon subconscious rules of thumb. If a doctor jumps to a conclusion, however, he or she might seek clues and only consider results that confirm that initial diagnosis, ignoring information that points in a different direction. For example, a middle aged woman comes to an ER very anxious and sweaty complaining she is having breathing trouble. She asks many questions, restlessly churns on the stretcher, and describes a recent stressful divorce. Easy diagnosis: Anxiety. Wrong! Heart attack. The doctor ignored subtle electrocardiogram abnormalities since it contradicted the initial conclusion that she was simply stressed out.

- **Distraction and chaos**: When a doctor or other practitioner is overwhelmed during a chaotic and busy emergency room shift, it is easy to jump to conclusions (known as premature closure, ie choosing the first reasonable diagnosis that comes to mind) or to have a "brain cramp" and overlook usually obvious clues and hints. Consider the "Brain Cramp" case published in a past issue of *Annals of Emergency Medicine*. Dr. Paul Yee describes his experience as follows:

"...being a neophyte emergency physician, I quickly realized I was in over my head... was up to my eyeballs with a couple of chest pains and abdominal pains, a few weak and dizzies, and plenty of walking wounded with various fractures and lacerations crowding the triage hallway... A leftover patient from the night shift had low blood pressure. Mr. X, who was never signed over to me, was an elderly man who presented with severe back pain that was diagnosed by the previous emergency physician as muscular in origin."

Dr. Yee goes on to describe how he agreed to discharge this man despite low blood pressure. The elderly man was wheeled back into the emergency department a few hours later – this time he was dead! Dr. Yee realized too late that the man's severe back pain and low blood pressure equaled a ruptured aneurysm of the aorta. This simple equation that all physicians are taught went right over Dr.

Yee's head as he suffered his "brain cramp" from mental fatigue during an overwhelming and chaotic emergency room shift.

- **Attitude bias**: Jumping to diagnostic conclusions based upon ageism, personality bias or "annoying" patient behaviors is sadly common. "This demented old fart shouldn't be in the ER taking time away from really sick people," or "He's just a drug seeker" or "That whining woman (with the heart attack) is a nervous wreck" so therefore doctors might dismiss their ailment as unimportant. Attitude bias can lead to outright misdiagnosis as well.

- **Overreliance on tests**: This category includes forgetting to check on results; misinterpretation of a test such as CT scan or electrocardiogram by an ER doctor, student or radiologist; ordering the wrong tests based upon incorrect first diagnostic impressions; and not considering the condition of the patient as greater priority over "normal" test results.

  Sometimes test-overkill occurs because doctors no longer trust their basic clinical reasoning and decision-making. A case report by Dr. Steven Horowitz that appeared in *Journal of American Medical Association: Internal Medicine* illustrates a testing-gone-wild approach to medical care that his sister experienced. Dr. Horowitz's healthy 65-year-old sister became disoriented with memory difficulties while at a friend's funeral. Dr. Horowitz, a neurologist, quickly recognized his sister suffered a temporary episode of transient global amnesia. He spoke to the emergency room doctor and predicted his sister would be recovered within several hours. She did return to normal seven hours later, but not before undergoing MRI's, angiograms, heart tests and a smorgasbord of blood tests. Final tab: $42,000! Couldn't they simply monitor her a few hours based upon the advice of her brother, Dr. Horowitz?

- **Overconfidence:** Charles Darwin is credited with writing "Ignorance more frequently begets confidence than does knowledge." I propose a corollary to this: Patients expect certainty from their healthcare providers. This can pressure an ER doctor into showing a façade of confidence and certainty even when, as is often the case, the diagnosis is unclear. The result: false reassurance that all is okay since nothing showed up on testing. In truth, a discussion about most likely diagnoses and a watch-and-wait approach for improvement or deterioration would be more prudent when uncertainty prevails in a person who is not feeling any better.

- **Very early presentation** of diseases can be elusive and misleading. Appendicitis, heart attack, TIA or stroke, for example, can be vague, confusing, and hard for any doctor to correctly diagnose very early on. Another example: electrocardiograms are frequently fairly normal in the early stages of a heart attack.
- **Unusual (atypical) symptoms** that occur uncommonly in any disease, especially in the elderly, can stump doctors. A common example: pneumonia in an elderly woman who has no fever or cough.

Testing Heresy: Reasons to Lose Faith in the Power of High-Tech Medical Tests

Ordering avoidable tests and treatments is an excuse, not a solution. Doctors often use these tactics as substitute for a thorough medical history and physical examination, meaningful communication, useful and practical patient education, reassurance and hand-holding. Ten-minute patient encounters no longer allow for these artful and caring approaches to diagnosis and treatment. Writing prescriptions or ordering tests are quick tasks that fit neatly into the fleeting, modern-day patient encounter. Tests and prescriptions also placate patients and serve to stifle insightful questioning by patients. "Let's wait to see what the test shows" or "Let's try this medication and see how you respond" are apt abrupt endings to patient encounters.

Why are doctors so test-happy? Several factors come into play. First, when technology is available, they use it. The United States boasts nearly 3 times as many MRI machines than average among industrialized nations. And doctors are trained to order, to probe and to investigate during their residency. Second, patients have been conditioned to expect quick answers and certainty, thus they demand more tests. This is a quintessential example of "Be careful of what you ask for you may get it." Third, doctors are highly motivated to test and treat, or risk getting sued for missing a diagnosis. A recent survey published in the *Archives of Internal Medicine* found

91 percent of doctors said they order avoidable tests and procedures to insulate themselves from lawsuits—a sobering statistic! Another powerful incentive to ordering more is financial gain. When doctors and hospitals generate higher income with more tests and procedures, even subconsciously, it is easy to rationalize more as being better.

According to a *New York Times* investigation published in 2012, the Office of Inspector General at the Health and Human Services Department sent a letter to emergency physicians nationwide requesting information about the practice of ordering unnecessary tests for financial gain.

Tests are Inherently Imperfect and Inaccurate

An emergency room doctor confessed to his patient uncertainty about the cause for her abdominal pain. "But didn't that blood test and ultrasound check for appendicitis?" she asked with a puzzled and pained look.

The physician surely took the correct approach by explaining to the patient that tests only provide clues to the possible presence or absence of disease. What is more important is how the patient feels, if there is improvement or deterioration over a few hours, and whether the physical examination shows continued cause for concern. Diagnosis must be a joint effort between both doctor and patient.

The doctor explained they had reached a key juncture: Should they proceed with a riskier test like CT scan which could be more accurate but causes significant radiation exposure and has intravenous contrast dye dangers? Or would it be reasonable to try sending her home since she felt a bit better after getting intravenous fluids? At home, she would still need to be vigilant and get quick follow up care, particularly if her condition went south. The more accurate CT scan can still miss the diagnosis of appendicitis as much as 10 percent of the time.

Some additional examples of inherently imperfect tests include:

- Colonoscopy done even by an experienced doctor can miss cancer in about 3 in 100 patients. And this test involves placing a scope *inside* the colon to look for disease!
- Exercise stress testing for heart disease is known to be less accurate in women under age 50. One way to improve accuracy of any

test is based upon the scientific principle called **Bayes' Theorem.** Simply stated: The more likely someone is to have a disease, the more accurate will be tests to check for that disease. Consider two people having some chest pain symptoms: An abnormal heart stress test in a 50-year old smoker with diabetes and high blood pressure is more likely to be true heart disease than a "positive" stress test in a healthy athlete of the same age.

- Ultrasound done in adults to diagnose appendicitis is *inaccurate* 15 percent of the time, on average, and can be far less reliable based upon how bloated the patient is and how experienced and skilled the ultrasound technician is.
- D-dimer is a blood test used in emergency rooms to exclude the serious diagnosis of pulmonary embolism, a blood clot in the lung. Studies have described its *inaccuracy* in older adults. A past study found the D-dimer blood test could reliably exclude the diagnosis of lung clot in 60 percent of patients younger than 40 years, but only ruled out this diagnosis in 5 percent of folks older than age 80 years. Risk factors for clots, the condition of the patient, and kidney function considerations must also be weighed in making an accurate diagnosis.

Useless Tests

When a doctor utters phrases such as "Just to be sure" or "just in case" or "Let's see if anything shows up" then I suggest you leap off the stretcher and run as fast as you can! These comments suggest that test the doctor plans to order is more for the doctor's benefit than the patient's well being. Allow me to complete the doctor's thought process when using these phrases: "Just in case... *I get sued*" and "Just to be sure... *my ass is covered.*"

A useless test is one that has little chance for providing any new or actionable information. It is unlikely to change the treatment plan, particularly when stakes are low and serious illness is unlikely in a patient who is not terribly ill. Several prestigious medical organizations have launched programs to encourage doctors to choose tests and treatments wisely and reduce testing or therapies that offer little benefit but significant risk.

Following are several varieties of useless tests:

Poor Choice of Test: This test type offers low accuracy to diagnose the illness in question. For instance, as mentioned, a CT scan will miss up to 80 percent of strokes in those patients experiencing only severe dizziness – so why not go directly to more accurate MRI testing if stroke is a likely diagnosis?

Will Not Change Treatment Plan: Some all too common examples include x-rays of an injured toe when taping the toes is the treatment whether bruised or broken. Sinus x-rays tend to offer little extra information for diagnosing acute sinusitis. Skull x-rays are rarely helpful, particularly in minor head trauma in which CT scanning is also overused and often avoidable. When a doctor orders an x-ray — or a CT scan or MRI —of your back after you wrenched your back lifting the sofa, the Choosing Wisely and Less is More quality care campaigns would advocate that you politely refuse the offer for imaging. Back imaging is not recommended for about 12 weeks if there is no improvement. Early testing should be done only for progressive pain and disability or with red flag signs of serious diseases like cancer.

Barking Up the Wrong Tree: You arrive at the emergency room with vague upper abdominal pains. The ER doctor orders an ultrasound of the abdomen to check for gallstones and reports the good news: it was normal so you can go home and take antacids. Problem: It was heart disease that caused the abdominal symptoms. Conversely, you undergo an electrocardiogram for your vague chest pains. The EKG is normal so you are quickly sent home. Problem: a serious gallbladder attack is what caused the chest discomfort. That doctor looked for disease in all the wrong places so testing would, of course, prove to be normal. He ignored the basic tenet that chest problems can cause abdominal pain and abdominal ailments often cause chest discomfort. In these situations experience and "index of suspicion" prove valuable for correct diagnosis.

Defensive Medicine at Play: This category describes the "just in case" tests (or treatments) that have as a goal to protect that doctor from potential lawsuits, not what is truly in the best interest of the patient. This type of useless testing is pervasive in medical practice (survey found 91% of doctors admit doing this). The only way around it: Ask the ordering doctor if the test in question is truly needed or can it wait. Ask if life or limb is at stake. Tell your treating doctor you are not interested in defensive medicine testing and will be happy to give things time to improve if life or death is not immediately at stake. If you make the decision to forego an iffy test or treatment many doctors will be thrilled and relieved. Others will feel absolved of guilt should a bad outcome occur and will document that "patient refused CT scan." Ultimately, you as patient must make the final decision how much risk and expense is worth undergoing based upon how sick you might be and if life is imperiled.

Misinterpreted Tests

Those who interpret tests are as imperfect as the tests themselves. Who might read an x-ray, CT scan or electrocardiogram in the emergency room? Doctors, nurse practitioners, doctors-in-training, and students often read results before a specialist is available to give an official reading.

Previous studies have found that up to 16 percent of x-rays and a staggering 33 percent of CT scans are misread in emergency departments, with many errors resulting in bad consequences. Even when CT scans are digitally transmitted on computer to a radiologist, digital readings tend to be less accurate than actual printed films. As technology improves this may become a moot point.

Electrocardiograms fair a little better. A 2006 study showed that one in eight EKGs read by emergency department personnel were misinterpreted. Accuracy tends to go way down in the absence of chest pain as a major complaint. In fact, the initial EKG in heart attack sufferers does not show clear evidence of impending heart damage in as many as 75 percent of cases.

X-rays and EKGs can be visually misread. Blood tests can simply be misinterpreted. For instance, a normal white blood cell count (measure of infection or inflammation) might be reassuring to an inexperienced doctor, but it is no comfort to a patient with severe, progressive abdominal pain. A seasoned medical professional understands that normal white blood cell count does *not* exclude appendicitis in this scenario, particularly in older folks who don't follow textbook rules.

Nefarious Reasons to Order Tests in ERs and Hospitals

As mentioned above, a 2012 New York Times investigation discussed the concerns nationwide that hospitals and emergency rooms are pressuring doctors to order more tests to generate higher income for the hospital. At times, the doctor's salary and job security are dependent upon how much money they generate for the hospital.

In addition, there have been reports that doctors will go along with needless tests and treatments so they can get a higher score on patient satisfaction surveys. Hospitals have implemented these tools across the country to improve public relations, but a doctor's job might be imperiled if patients are not placated, even if that doctor tries to practice quality care by deferring on avoidable and risky tests or treatments.

Tips to Renew Your Faith in Tests and Avoid their Pitfalls

Tests can be vital in helping doctors make difficult diagnoses. But they can also provide misleading information, leading to unnecessary worry and risky procedures. Many tests expose people to radiation as well – significant amounts! (see page 93, CT Scan Radiation Exposure Amounts)

Imaging tests such as CT scan or MRI often find what are called "incidentalomas." As discussed earlier, these are shadows, spots, cysts or masses that are found incidentally and were not the reason for ordering the test. They are usually harmless and represent normal variation in our bodies, imperfect imaging shadows or over-reading by radiologists, and harmless cysts (as in the case discussed earlier of the woman who had her kidney removed). These incidentalomas rarely prove to be serious diseases. Interestingly, there is growing controversy as to whether *actual* cancers can be left alone and monitored if they cause no symptoms. Some cancers are slow-growing and will never affect the individual in his or her natural lifetime; some cancers might regress and never cause trouble so finding them is considered by some experts to be over-diagnosis. Monitoring these small, silent masses for growth every few months might be prudent rather than undergoing dangerous biopsies or surgery. It is surely difficult to do nothing when told a possible cancer may be lurking within, especially since medical science cannot yet accurately determine which masses are harmless and which might suddenly spread.

What is most puzzling is people's reactions to discovering incidentalomas, as described well by Dr. Lisa Schwartz and colleagues in an *Archives of Internal Medicine* editorial. More often than not, people are subjected to weeks of anxiety about a so-called "abnormality" and undergo more and more risky tests. Sometimes, they agree to biopsies and even major surgery. Diagnosis: Benign. Nothing. Nada. Oops. Incidentaloma. Patient reaction: Thankful. Praise. Thank God for high-tech imaging. Let's do more. Schwartz and colleagues explain that kidney cancer diagnoses have doubled since 1975 but the death rate is the same. Catching the cancer earlier with fancy technology doesn't necessarily mean a life saved. Many of these cancers would never have shown up if the person dies of other causes before the kidney cancer reared its ugly head.

While it may be difficult to digest since we still know so little, some cancers do grow slowly and pose little or no risk. For instance, the National Lung Screening Trial has shown that nearly 1 in 5 lung cancers detected by CT scan screening appeared to be indolent, meaning slow-growing and possibly harmless.

As another example of over-diagnosis, think about how often women are subjected to suspicious shadows, spots or cysts on their screening mammograms and undergo biopsies after weeks of worry. "Thank God for testing," they proclaim, while exhaling after weeks of breath-holding. Should they be thankful or angry for over-diagnosis and over-testing?

You as patient and medical care consumer must act as the final judge of whether or not to undergo risky tests. Leave it up to the doctor and you will usually end up getting the tests. First step: do your own research and ask probing questions. Then follow this general guide:

1. **How sick am I?** If you have a potentially life-threatening illness then clearly the benefit scale gets weighted more heavily to go forward with riskier testing like CT scans, angiograms, MRI with dye, nuclear medicine tests, and procedures like biopsies or surgery. Examples include worst-ever abdominal pain; thunderclap headache; severe, unexplained shortness of breath; unfamiliar

chest pains that stop your activities of daily living; unexplained fainting; worst-ever back pain that stops you in your tracks; and many others. Clearly, having other chronic illnesses like heart disease, diabetes, cancer etc. puts you at risk for a more serious ailment and should lower the threshold for proceeding with testing. On the other side of the coin, a migraine headache in a healthy adult does not always justify a CT scan of the brain. Adults with no risk factors for a clot in the lung do not always need to undergo a CT scan of the lungs for an episode of mild shortness of breath.

2. **Can testing wait?** Assuming imminent life or death is off the table, ask the emergency doctor what would likely happen if you simply waited a day or two to see your family doctor and get testing then, if needed. This is a crucial question to cut through the defensive medicine fog. If the doctor says, "Sure, no problem, I will just chart that you refused the test" or "Sure, it can wait if you want to" then clearly you have your answer. Some ER doctors, however, are obsessively test-happy out of fear of missing a serious illness, or due to pressure to generate more hospital revenue. This type of doctor might insist on testing even though life or limb are likely not at risk. If you suspect this is the case, ask for another doctor's opinion before you decide. It can be your trusted family doctor or the physician in charge of the emergency department. But you must make it clear that you are not interested in "just in case" tests.

   Note: Specialists will usually err on the side of ordering *more* tests or procedures.

3. **Play the defensive medicine card.** At this point, if a doctor insists on getting a questionable test without logical explanations why, you might be forced to say it loud and clear that you only want the best care, not worthless and risky tests that will not help you.

4. **Am I feeling better?** Discuss with the emergency doctor first trying simpler and safer treatments and tests before moving to the risky stuff. For example, severe right-sided back pain in a healthy 50-year old – maybe a wrenched back, maybe a kidney stone? Try intravenous fluids, pain medicine, a urine test for blood, an

ultrasound of the kidneys, and tincture of time. If you are much better then you can get follow up with your family doctor for further evaluation. No need to rush into CT scans and contrast dye tests if you feel better within a few hours. Sometimes, several hours of observation and simple treatments like intravenous fluids are all that is required to distinguish serious from self-improving sickness.

5. **Benefits versus risks?** If it seems like a riskier test is in the cards, ask if *safer* alternatives can be tried first to clinch the diagnosis. Then discuss what the risky test or procedure will find or exclude from a list of possible diagnoses the doctor lists for you. What are the worst risks of the test? What are the most common risks? How much radiation will you be exposed to? How accurate is that test in detecting or excluding the disease in question? Will the result alter the likely treatment plan?

Key Points to Remember

- Never accept any test or treatment that is ordered before an ER medical provider sees you, takes a medical history, examines you, and discusses reasons for testing and benefits versus risks. That doctor, nurse practitioner or physician assistant should then answer your questions. Exception: simple tests like basic blood work might be ordered at triage to expedite the ER visit.
- Avoid the "whatever you say, doc" attitude to your care. Ultimately, you must be the gatekeeper for deciding to undergo a test or not. Politely decline the iffy and unnecessary ones. Listen to your body. If you are improving then simple tests and treatments are best. If you feel seriously ill with little improvement, accepting riskier tests and treatments might be appropriate. Specialist consultations are also beneficial for progressive acute illness or for people with several complex, chronic ailments.
- Chant the "**Is it safe**?" mantra every time tests or treatments are being discussed. While the question had very different meaning in the movie *Marathon Man* as Laurence Olivier relentlessly repeated the phrase to Dustin Hoffman's character, the importance of asking this question in the emergency room setting is clear.

- If in doubt about the need for risky tests, feel free to ask for other opinions – a specialist consultation, family doctor, relative, ER nurse, or the ER physician-in-charge. Caveat: Specialists do tend to order more, rather than fewer, tests. Clarify that you only want testing if truly needed, not for less serious ailments or just in case.
- Never assume no news is good news. Be sure any tests you undergo are carefully reviewed by the ER doctor and specialist (Radiologist, for example) and results are explained to you in easy to understand terms.
- Doctors often take cues from patients to determine how much testing the patient expects. If you start naming tests your friends had last month then you may end up getting the million dollar workup as well, whether or not it is truly helpful.
- Be wary of tests ordered in primary care and specialist offices or urgent care centers when they are done in-house. These tests generate extra income for that practice so you want to be cautious that motives are pure and the tests are truly needed. Ask the ordering doctor or provider the questions discussed above to help determine that.
- Reminder: Tests and procedures sometimes lead to more questions than answers. They are inherently inaccurate and imperfect. Technology does not equal certainty. In our quest for certainty, patients must submit to the reality that there is no certainty. More and more tests and procedures often lead to more and more trouble – not more certainty.
- Imperfections aside, test results are only as good as the equipment used, the technician or lab performing the test, and the specialist interpreting the result. Be wary of traveling screening trucks or storefront screening discounts since the quality of tests – and thus their reliability – may be subpar.
- Radiation risk from medical tests and procedures remains in the background like chatter in a crowded room: the risks are present but not really paid much mind. Following are a few low doses of enlightenment:

* Between 1998 and 2007 there was a tripling of the number of CT scans and MRIs done for injuries. Only a tiny fraction of these tests yield significant findings. Many trauma centers routinely perform whole-body CT scans on even mild to moderately injured patients!

* Estimates suggest that one to two percent of all cancers in the United States and United Kingdom are now associated with CT scan radiation exposure.

* Getting imaging studies can increase by several hours an emergency room visit and may contribute to overcrowding, chaos and errors in that setting.

* Teaching hospitals, in general, are more likely to perform imaging and other tests or procedures than are community hospitals.

* One in 14 emergency department patients underwent a head CT scan and 1 in 400 had a head MRI, according to recent reports. Increasing age was the strongest predictor of undergoing these tests. To illustrate overuse, studies have shown that imaging for headaches finds significant abnormalities only 1 to 3 percent of the time. If the tests are okay 97 to 99 percent of the time then surely some of these tests could have been avoided with careful evaluation and close medical follow up.

* Each day about 20,000 CT scans are performed in the United States, exposing each person to the equivalent of between 30 and 400 chest x-rays in one fell swoop!

* Fear of lawsuits may account for 1 in 5 imaging tests doctors order, according to one study.

* The agency that oversees Medicare and Medicaid looked at regions of the United States with pockets of higher imaging use and concluded those areas do *not* have better outcomes in patient care.

* CT scans use much higher doses of radiation than regular x-rays. For example, a CT scan of the chest delivers about 100 times the dose of radiation that a simple chest x-ray does! It

gets worse. Survivors of the Hiroshima and Nagasaki atomic bombs were found to suffer an increased cancer risk. The dose of radiation exposure they sustained was not much different than many modern day CT scan tests as explained in the sidebar on radiation risk.

A Few More Helpful Suggestions

In an ideal situation, patients should be informed about specific radiation exposure risks before any imaging test or procedure. There should be a required consent form that must be signed specifying the approximate dose of radiation exposure and other risks such as kidney damage from intravenous contrast dye. California has recently enacted a law requiring imaging facilities to report radiation doses to patients and their doctors. This law is a first step.

Another suggestion is the **Radiation Record**: All people should carry a card or digital record of any and all radiation tests they undergo from birth, similar to an immunization record. Radiation exposure risk is cumulative throughout a lifetime so exposure amounts should be considered by every patient and doctor. Each and every order for imaging should consider this radiation record. A good place for people to begin to learn about imaging tests and procedures and their risks is on the American College of Radiology website: http://www.radiologyinfo.org/.

Newer scanning machines boast lower radiation doses for equal or better quality images. Find out if the scanner you will be rolled into is the latest techno-gadget or yesterday's news – like last year's model of smartphone.

Watch-and-wait should be the new testing mantra. A waiting period of a few hours to a couple of days should be the standard for all imaging studies or risky procedures when illness is not imminently life-threatening.

Do not allow imaging to substitute for a doctor performing a thorough history and physical examination, though many doctors have lost the art and knowledge required to do this well. Do not allow time constraints, ER crowding and need for rapid-fire stretcher turnover to squash a wise watch-and-wait approach in situations where life and death are not imminent. A few hours of simple tests, safe treatments and observation in the emergency room can heal many ailments.

CT Scan Radiation Exposure Amounts (mSv units) and Equivalent Number of Plain x-rays

CT Scan or x-ray Type	Approx. Radiation Dose (mSv)	Approx. # Regular x-rays Equivalent
Atom Bomb Hiroshima and Nagasaki causing increased cancer risk	**10 to 100 mSv**	--------
Plain Chest x-ray	**0.1 mSv**	--------
Chest CT Scan	8 mSv	80 – 110 x-rays
Chest, Suspected Lung Clot	10 mSv	100 – 130 x-rays
Heart Angiogram CT Scan	22 mSv	200 – 300 x-rays
Brain CT Scan for Stroke	14 mSv	100 – 200 x-rays
Abdomen/Pelvis CT Scan	15 to 30 mSv	200 to 400 x-rays

DANGER 5. TREATMENTS WORSE THAN THE DISEASE

"Don't just do something... stand there!"

Dr. Jerry Hoffman, UCLA (quipped during personal communication about overtreatment in medical care)

"The great secret known to internists, but still hidden from the general public... is that most things get better by themselves. Most things, in fact, are better by morning."

Lewis Thomas, physician, essayist, medical researcher

"Treatment" is a magical word. It is surely a sweet and soothing sound after the hammer of sickness batters and bruises one's body. "Treatment" has a reassuring, hopeful ring that all can be well again and body balance can be restored. In truth, a treatment is no guarantee of cure. Many treatments are dubious and offer false promises at best (Laetrile for cancer, anyone?), dangerous side effects, and even serious risks. Today's "miracle" medical procedures and impressive scientific articles are often tainted by trendy over-use, focus on lab data and numbers rather than patient wishes and actual benefit, as well as hidden motives such as financial profits. Following are several examples – old and new – of wonder treatments gone awfully wrong. It is always wise to view treatments with healthy skepticism until benefits are explained and clearly outweigh risks. It is vitally important to consider treatments guilty until proven innocent, so to speak, especially in frail older folks who have decreased ability to manage body insults and stressors. Sadly, comedienne Joan Rivers' tragic death is a reminder that even simple procedures are not harmless, especially as we age. Read on and draw your own conclusions.

Dr Antonio Moniz was a little-known Portuguese neurologist with big ideas. He had a hand in the development of contrast dye called Thorotrast which helped early Twentieth-Century doctors get a look at blood vessels in the brain - an amazing innovation and variation of angiograms commonly used today with CT scans and MRIs. But that did not win him a Nobel Prize. He reportedly was nominated for a Nobel Prize for his innovations in visualization of brain blood vessels, a technique called cerebral angiography. He finally did win the coveted Nobel Prize for innovative brain surgeries for diseases that had no available treatments. His surgical technique evolved over time. Initially, he would drill holes into the skull and inject an alcohol solution into a specific area of the brain. Soon Dr. Moniz used more refined technique and simply sliced possibly diseased connections with a fine wire in exactly the correct part of the brain. He soon proclaimed wonderful results. Doctors around the world adopted this novel and unique treatment for which Dr. Moniz would win the 1949 Nobel Prize for Medicine. The diseases his surgical procedures treated were schizophrenia, anxiety and depression. The part of the brain he operated upon: frontal lobe. The name of the surgical innovation worthy of this grand prize: prefrontal leucotomy, later renamed "Lobotomy" by American neurologist Walter Freeman. Freeman also promoted this "innovative" treatment and later noted, "Every patient probably loses something by this operation, some spontaneity, some sparkle, some flavor of the personality." And the novel Thorotrast dye used in up to 10 million patients worldwide during the 1930's and 1940's - that was proven to increase cancer risk by a factor of 10 to 100 times! The dye's dangerous alpha radiation would remain inside patients for decades, all in the interest of doctors getting good x-ray images of blood vessels.

Lesson: Just because a disease has no effective treatments, does not mean the latest newfangled treatment or procedure is helpful, safe and in the best interest of the patient. Lobotomy may well go down in history as the most extreme example of a treatment far worse than the disease! Thorazine, the first antipsychotic medication, did not become available until the 1950's at which time most doctors stopped using the barbaric, award-winning lobotomy procedure. Always wait for new treatments (or new uses for older treatments) to be proven safe and effective.

Interestingly, Dr. Moniz reportedly was shot by one of his schizophrenic patients in 1949. It is safe to say he should have scheduled that patient for lobotomy surgery sooner.

Trephining: Barbaric or Life-saving?

Perhaps the first known surgical procedure ever used by man was called trephining. Those who performed this procedure drilled or scraped holes into someone's skull until the brain covering was exposed – while the patient was awake! Barbaric? But surgeons continue to perform this operation today. Back then the procedure was done using coarse instruments on the cold, hard ground, and 'treated' headaches, epilepsy and psychiatric disease as well as close-combat head injuries. Headache, epilepsy and mental illness are hardly good risk versus benefit uses of such a dangerous procedure. Modern-day surgeons use the more refined version of trephination – in a sterile operating room—and drill Burr holes only for life-threatening ailments like brain bleeding or swelling. The lesson learned: relatively simple problems rarely warrant highly risky solutions. Potentially dangerous procedures and treatments should be reserved for life or death illnesses after a careful analysis of whether benefit has been scientifically proven.

Swan-Ganz Catheters: Miracle Medical Device or Useless Gadget?

Dr. Werner Forssmann was a newly minted German doctor in 1929 when he made history in an unusual way. One workday he inserted a long, pencil-thin tube into his *own* arm vein and threaded it through until it reached his heart. He then walked over to an x-ray machine and got an image of the catheter tip resting in his right atrium heart chamber. Forssmann proved that the heart could be 'touched' and it won him a Nobel Prize for Medicine in 1956. This ultimately led to the routine use of balloon-tipped catheters being inserted deeper into the heart, developed in 1970 by Drs. Swan and Ganz. These catheters were inserted into most critically ill patients for the next two decades since they arguably provided key information about how the heart and circulatory system were functioning. The goal was to help guide proper therapy using information gleaned from the device, believed to be a medical marvel and a window into the wondrous workings of the heart while the patient rested in a sedative-induced soporific haze.

As Dr. William Heberden aptly claimed in the 18th Century: "New medicines, and new methods of cures, always work miracles... for a while." How true this statement was for the fate of the Swan-Ganz catheter. When the novelty and glee of this medical Tinker-toy faded, doctors realized that critically-ill patients fared better when they did *not* get this catheter inserted in their heart through a neck or chest vein. Those with the catheter died in greater numbers. This "miracle" method of cure did, fortunately, last just a relatively short while. The lesson learned: Just because we could tinker with and "touch" the heart in live patients, does not mean people actually benefited from the latest medical gizmo.

Some concerns with medical treatments:

1. Questionable medical studies: Studies done to show treatments are both effective and safe are often paid for by companies with an interest in good outcomes. These studies exclude frail elderly so any true benefits may not apply to seniors who take many other medications, have reduced kidney function and several chronic ailments, and whose bodies are in delicate balance. Expert analyses have also found understating of side effects and non-publication of studies showing no benefit to treatments. Aggressive marketing of the arthritis drug, Vioxx, went on unabated despite mounting evidence of the increased heart attack risk for Vioxx users. This pain medication became a billion dollar blockbuster drug before it was taken off the market due to safety concerns.
2. Doctors frequently recommend treatments and tests based upon expert opinion guidelines published by prestigious medical organizations and respected experts in that specialty. Recent studies and discussion in the medical literature voice great concern about the validity of those guidelines upon which doctors base crucial medical care decisions. For instance, a recent *Archives of Internal Medicine* study on conflicts of interest in cardiovascular practice

guidelines found many disturbing revelations. More than half of the "expert" authors who helped develop guidelines for practicing doctors to follow in caring for heart patients had significant conflicts of interest such as owning stock in a medical device company or serving as paid promotional speaker for a pharmaceutical or device manufacturer. What's more, reports show nearly half of all recent heart guidelines are based only on weak evidence called "expert opinion," rather than objective randomized clinical studies. Even the expert specialty societies that publish treatment recommendations have sold out and receive millions of dollars from industries that produce drugs and medical devices! Finally, expert guidelines supposedly set the standard of medical care but rarely consider a patient preference approach to care. These recommendations are one size fits all and fail to consider differences in needs and goals among individual patients.

3. The medical establishment has every reason to turn every problem into a nail when they earn lots of money selling hammers. Many experts have questioned the ever-expanding list of those who are "sick" and need a drug treatment or procedure. A "weak bladder" from aging is now "overactive bladder" and seems to require drug treatment. The "diseases" of pre-diabetes and pre-hypertension have now transformed millions of previously normal folks into life-long pill-takers who suffer from early, chronic illness. Now big pharmaceutical companies have created "Low-T" in aging men with shrinking testosterone levels. Apparently we have not learned much from the low estrogen fad of yesteryear, treatment of which turned out to increase cancer and heart disease risks significantly. Many questions remain about the safety of testosterone replacement in men. And your cholesterol level – apparently it can never be low enough for you to be safe so everybody needs a statin drug (more on statins below).

Patients must have healthy skepticism about any guidelines and recommendations their doctor suggests if it does not make sense to you as health consumer, or if the recommendation is not in keeping with personal needs and goals.

Let us now consider some *modern-day* examples of treatments that might be worse than the disease:

Tight Diabetes Control: Better High than Low?

If you have always believed that tight blood sugar control in all diabetics makes good sense and is advocated purely for the good of the patients, sorry to burst your bubble. It's complicated. The dizzying display of dozens of designer diabetes drugs surely plays a role. Dr. Sei Lee offers interesting insight into this issue in commentary published in May 2014 in the *Journal of the American Medical Association Internal Medicine*. Lee describes how the pharmaceutical industry has molded widely accepted beliefs that tight blood sugar control is always best and insulin or other drug treatments are the path to achieving that goal. Lee explains that in 2002, Aventis, the pharmaceutical company that manufactures a commonly-used type of designer insulin, teamed up with public relations firm Burson-Marsteller to successfully sway key organizations such as the American Diabetes Association and the National Committee for Quality Assurance to promote tighter and tighter blood sugar control. One such slogan, "Aim, Believe, Achieve" influenced both doctors and patients to strive for still lower blood sugars. Then in 2008, a major clinical study called ACCORD was stopped 17 months early because significantly more people died in the group getting *tighter* sugar control! Yet doctors continue to push tighter blood sugar control and frequent A1c blood tests as they are required to meet certain vague standards of performance measures. Sadly, these measures focus more on better lab numbers, not better individual patient care. And which patient group had the highest risk for emergency room visits and hospitalizations from low blood sugar? The elderly. The hospital admission rate for *low* blood sugar now exceeds that for *high* blood sugar in older adults, according to new research. Even though low blood sugar is a reversible illness, 1 in 5 older adults in this study hospitalized for low blood sugar died within a year.

Heart Disease Treatment – Two-Edged Sword

When doctors developed the technology to scrape open blockages in heart arteries and restore crucial blood flow, it seemed to be a miraculous treatment advance for heart disease. Specialists would thread a catheter through the leg artery into heart-feeding arteries and expand a balloon to force open the hardened plaque deposits formed from years of smoking and dietary indiscretions. First, cardiologists performed an angiogram in which contrast dye is injected into arteries then x-ray pictures helped to show well-defined outlines of heart-feeding arteries. Many arteries showed a "pinching in" or narrowing effect wherein the dye must squeeze through an artery with 50 percent or 70 percent or even 99 percent plaque-deposit blockage. Seemed straight forward enough to open those blockages and restore heart harmony. Nothing, however, is simple in medicine as regards the complex human body. Doctors then learned that fixed piles of plaque heaped up in a narrowed artery do *not* themselves cause heart attacks. It is *damage* to the plaque and inner lining of the heart artery, combined with a state of inflammation, which leads to a fully obstructing, sudden blood clot in that artery. This cuts off the blood supply to a portion of the heart, causing a heart attack. That 60 percent plaque blockage in an artery will not necessarily lead to a heart attack, nor will it necessarily cause trouble sooner than an artery only 30 percent blocked with fixed, hard plaque.

Then cardiologists developed stents that serve as metal tunnels to prop open arteries and help prevent the pesky problem of one-third of ballooned-open arteries re-obstructing within 30 days. Despite the ingenuity and high-tech advances, several key points warrant emphasis regarding getting treatments for heart disease:

- Help yourself avoid the need to undergo invasive heart procedures by taking control of your heart disease risk factors right now (see Chest Pain Chapter).
- Drs. Stergiopoulos and Brown performed an analysis of the best studies involving stent placement and their conclusions were published in 2012, in the *Archives of Internal Medicine*: Stent placement for stable heart disease with milder symptoms offers no benefit over treatment with medications for prevention of death, heart attack and angina. They also explain that the stenting procedure itself may cause heart attacks during the procedure in 5 to 30 percent of patients! A 2012 *New York Times* article by Nicholas Bakalar quotes Dr. Harlan Krumholz, Cardiologist and Professor

of Medicine at Yale University. Krumholz's wise words: "When people are making decisions, it's important to disclose to them that this procedure (stent) — outside of an emergency (heart attack) — is not known to be lifesaving or to prevent heart attacks," he said. "The vast majority of people who have this procedure have the expectation that it will help them live longer. That belief is out of alignment with the evidence."

- Dr. Eric Topol, renowned cardiologist and medical researcher, coined the term "**oculostenotic reflex**." This refers to the reflexive need doctors have to force open any blockage (stenosis) they see on an angiogram. Highly touted studies with names such as COURAGE showed no benefit doing invasive stents over simply taking medications for *stable* heart disease (does not apply to an acute heart attack). If you need further convincing that heart procedures are not always beneficial, the United States performs more than triple the number of balloon angioplasties, stents and bypass heart surgeries as compared with Canada. So Americans must be far more heart healthy? Wrong. There is little difference in heart disease deaths and disability between the high-procedure versus low-procedure countries.
- A recent study comparing heart bypass surgery (CABG) to only taking medications in patients suffering from heart failure showed little benefit for those undergoing the major and risky operation. Dr. Harlan Krumholz, Professor of Medicine at Yale University, once again was quoted in a *Journal of the American Medical Association* article in response to the findings of this study: "I'm trying to envision the patient where you sit down with him or her and say, 'We can treat you with medicine or open you up and get to the same place.' Which patient might say, 'I want to have my chest opened and face a possible risky recovery'?"
- The risk of major bleeding from heart procedures like angioplasty and stenting is significant and can be as high as 4 to 7 percent. What's more, there is a clear connection between serious bleeding during the procedure and future death. And blood transfusion

is needed in up to 16 percent of cases of bleeding from heart procedures.

- Angiograms to delineate blockages in heart arteries were found to show no artery disease in two-thirds of these procedures when done for less typical heart attack symptoms such as shortness of breath, or for those without clear symptoms but with high cholesterol and similar risk factors, according to one recent study. If two-thirds of angiograms were negative, perhaps the test is overused?

Statin Therapy for All?

"Statinization" of the planet sounds like a low-budget science fiction flick but it is, in fact, a real concern voiced by Dr. John Ioannidis, a Stanford University medical researcher, in his editorial published in the *Journal of the American Medical Association*, February 2014. He estimates that the new American Heart Association guidelines on heart disease risk assessment adds another 46 million people in the United States who would be eligible to take these potent cholesterol-lowering drugs with a doctor's recommendation and blessing. Globally, that translates into nearly 1 billion new statin users between ages 40 and 79 years. Why the fuss? Guidelines are now recommending statins like Lipitor, Crestor and Zocor for those who may have increased risk but who have never actually had heart disease or stroke. Numerous studies do show reduced death and disease in those with established heart disease or previous stroke who take statins. The risk-benefit decision may well tilt in favor of taking the drug for sicker, high-risk patients. What about healthier patients with mild to moderate risk for artery-blocking diseases? The evidence is quite weak for benefit in healthy folks with high cholesterol according to expert analysis by physicians. A group of researchers created insightful analysis of this topic on the NNT Group website, which offers the following sober explanation of risks and benefits for a healthy adult with mild to moderately high cholesterol who takes a statin drug:

Folks who took a statin drug daily for five years: 98 percent saw no benefit, 0 percent avoided death by taking the drug, 1.6 percent had a heart attack prevented and 0.4 percent had a stroke prevented. The harms: two percent developed diabetes, a serious chronic disease. About

10 percent experienced muscle damage and pain. Interestingly, a recent study found an association between statin drugs and joint injuries, thus limiting the very activity needed to help reduce cholesterol and inflammation. Moreover, the Mediterranean diet has been shown to reduce heart attacks and strokes by 30 percent, which beats the benefits of statin drugs. You as health consumer must decide if benefits of taking medication outweigh risks.

What's more concerning, there is reason to question the integrity of the so-called evidence of benefit for healthier adults taking statin drugs. With the new American Heart Association and American College of Cardiology heart disease guidelines, it has been widely reported that 8 of the 15 expert panelists had conflict-of-interest ties to medical companies that stand to benefit from more aggressive treatment. This tainted guidance is the best doctors have to work with to advise patients. Healthy skepticism is always wise. Also, the major drug study that got this over-treatment train rolling, called JUPITER, was quickly bashed by experts as being flawed in a big way, had suspicious patterns of results, and was overseen closely by the medical companies that stood to gain from positive results.

A Simple Procedure: Unintended Consequences

Soon after retirement an elderly man is stricken with Alzheimer's disease. His wife dutifully cares for him despite the emotional and physical toll that chips away at her soul and body night after night. Care questions begin to mount: Should he get cancer screening tests like colonoscopy? His cardiologist recommends he get his pacemaker battery changed since it was overdue. Why not? It involves just cutting the chest skin under anesthesia for a few short minutes. His family agreed to proceed but things did not go as planned. He awoke from anesthesia screaming, disoriented and swinging at nurses who came within arm's reach. His wife was called into the recovery room to help soothe him but to no avail. He plucked at his intravenous line and continued to swing at anything close by. His wife was deeply traumatized as she watched her husband of 50 years suffer, act violently, and hit bottom. A "simple" procedure turned into a major ordeal for the patient, caregiver and family. Frail elderly are delicate and have little ability to adapt or compensate to any outside stresses. This true personal experience that was published in the *Journal of the American Medical Association* in March 2014 by Dr. Marjorie Rosenthal illustrates how care decisions affect not only the patient, but also family members, especially those who undertake the caregiver role.

Tootsie's Story: When is it Time to Say, "Enough?"

Jennifer Bellot, PhD, an assistant professor at Thomas Jefferson University, describes how a "simple" dosing error in her grandmother's thyroid medication led to a cascade of deterioration in Tootsie's fragile state of health. The excess thyroid drug caused her delicately-balanced, failing heart to beat rapidly and irregularly. Doctors tried to 'zap' her heart back into normal rhythm and Tootsie soon developed kidney failure, pneumonia and anemia. Sadly, Tootsie spent her final days not at home in comforting presence of her family, as Bellot explains in her essay published by the Robert Wood Johnson Foundation:

> In the final five months of her life, Tootsie went home for a total of 2.5 days. In the meantime, she had at least six hospital admissions at two facilities that involved three intensive care stays, six visits to the emergency department, a cardiac catheterization, five units of blood, an upper endoscopy and a startling number of chest x-rays, EKGs and blood tests. She quickly became deconditioned and spent every day that she was not in the hospital as a resident of the adjoining nursing home, determined through therapy and exercise to regain her independence.

Tootsie clearly endured a great deal of high-tech medical treatments in her final few months of life with little gained from all the treatments modern medicine had to offer. Each person, as they near end of life, must decide at what point quality of life supersedes more and more aggressive treatment. Should Tootsie have declined the heart catheterization? Was the stomach endoscopy too much for her frail condition? And the pokes and prods that tormented Tootsie daily – when should those have been called off? These philosophical questions can only be answered by personal preferences, not medical tenets. The exception is the tenet, "First do no harm."

Lessons Learned from Treatments that are Worse than the Disease

There are several categories of treatments to consider when you find yourself suddenly ill on a hard stretcher:

(a) **Dangerous and unproven treatments**: The use of clot-dissolving drugs or Roto-rooter mechanical removal of clots that cause strokes falls squarely into this category. Although some patients get good results, there remains great skepticism about the quality of the major studies regarding safety and effectiveness. Many studies that have shown worse outcomes in treated patients have been downplayed. Many emergency physicians in recent years have refused to order this controversial treatment for their stroke patients (See also, Stroke Chapter).

(b) **Quite risky, but proven to be beneficial treatments**: An example of this type of treatment is clot-dissolving treatment for heart attack. This approach to treating a heart attack can be lifesaving for a massive heart attack. Because the risk for deadly bleeding is high, a mild heart attack may warrant more careful consideration and discussion of risks versus benefits. Incredibly, a 2015 analysis of over 250 risky procedures found 227 of these procedures to be high risk in those over age 65, according to a *Journal of the American Medical Association Surgery* article. A colon resection for cancer, for instance, has high death rates in the elderly. Of all procedures studied, 154 procedures had an in-hospital death rate of 6 percent in older adults! Even a one percent death rate is generally considered risky in any adult.

(c) **Possibly helpful with small gains but high daily costs**: These high costs come in the form of taking an expensive drug or potentially experiencing some of many possible side effects. Some medications may contribute to reduced quality of life. Several drugs require the inconvenience of periodic blood tests. These prescriptions, even when tolerated, require a daily commitment to take the drug for years. Treatment with statin drugs for mild to moderately high cholesterol in a person who never had heart disease or stroke is a perfect example, as described in detail above.

(d) **Very beneficial to many, but many side effects likely**: Chemotherapy for cancer and newer disease-modifying drugs for rheumatoid arthritis are just two examples appropriate to this category

Treatments in frail elders must always be viewed with suspicion since even so-called simple therapies can have devastating consequences in delicate elders. The domino effect of one complication followed by another can rob these folks of remaining quality of life in their final days.

DANGER 6. RISKS OF HOSPITALIZATION: WILTING WHILE UNDER CARE

Hospitals can be a haven for the sick, or a living hell. Emergency rooms, which often serve as the gateway into hospitals, also provide the best of care and the worst of care for sick older adults. That wise adage "The hospital is the worst place to be when you are sick" is surely true. What could possibly go wrong in a hospital with such nice nurses and all that fancy technology? Read on and you will get a bitter dose of reality about the many potential harms of in-hospital care, along with tips to help avoid those pitfalls.

When Death is Personal

A 69 year old woman suddenly feels palpitations and difficulty breathing. The emergency room doctor at a prestigious teaching hospital diagnoses her with atrial fibrillation, a potentially dangerous irregular heart rhythm. Her cardiologist admits her into the hospital and fills her veins with blood-thinning medication to prevent a clot from forming inside the heart. With no available bed, she remains in the crowded emergency room – noise, hard stretcher, bright lights and all. Because of the delay in getting her to a medical floor, her echocardiogram is delayed. If all is ok on that ultrasound test of the heart, then doctors would literally shock her heart back into normal rhythm. The weekend was now upon them and the new plan was simple: she would remain on blood thinners in the hospital all weekend until the new week arrived. But as is often the case in hospitals, things did not go as planned.

Disaster struck to shatter the quiet of a slow Saturday in the hospital. That lady suddenly experienced numbness on one side of her body. She could not move her arm or leg. A large blood clot had formed in her heart and traveled to block off flow in a brain-feeding artery. A neurosurgeon was available at this teaching hospital and attempted to remove the blood clot using a roto-rooter-type medical device. This dangerous procedure would hopefully return nutrient and blood flow to her brain and stop the stroke in its tracks. Sadly, this as yet unproven treatment tore through the major artery, leading to hemorrhage inside her brain – the most dreaded of complications since she was on blood thinners. Death loomed near as she lay in an intensive care unit on a breathing machine without signs of improvement.

The preceding true story is based upon an essay written by Dr. John Maa, Assistant Professor of Surgery, University of California at San Francisco. It was published in the New England Journal of Medicine in 2011. That 69 year old woman was his mother. In the end, life support was withdrawn about 100 hours after she walked into the hospital expecting world-class care.

Dr. Maa wondered if the delays in care – getting a floor bed, an echo-cardiogram and shock treatment to her heart – might have contributed to this tragic outcome. Perhaps closer monitoring of her blood-thinning treatment could have prevented that deadly clot from forming in her heart.

Dr. Maa makes several disturbing and relevant observations in his essay:

> *"Boarding"(holding) admitted patients in emergency department exam rooms and corridors for extended periods has become so commonplace that it is accepted as the norm, particularly in large urban hospitals. But a crowded ED (emergency room) is more than a nuisance; it is a threat both to individual patients and to overall public health.*
>
> *Crowded emergency rooms are only one part of the problem. Inefficient hospital operations are another. Death, disease, and injury occur around the clock, but many hospitals still operate the majority of their services only 5 days a week. A growing number of specialists are either refusing to take after-hours call or demanding payments for doing so. After-hours and weekend gaps in coverage have real consequences; death rates from heart attacks and similar serious conditions are higher on weekends compared to weekdays.*

Joe's Story

What is the harm in "playing it safe" and sending an elderly person to the hospital for care?

Joe's story will shed light on just a few of the hidden dangers lurking in all ER's and hospitals. It's a jungle *in* there!

Joe was a tobacco farmer from the South when he wore a younger man's clothes. He was also known to puff on a few hand-rolled cigarettes in his day. Joe never acknowledged his "baggy heart" might have been connected to his decades of tobacco indulgences. "It's from old age," Joe always insisted. Whatever the cause, he now suffered from bouts of water in his lungs. An occasional dietary indiscretion like ham during holiday season, or a run-of-the-mill bad heart day, would tip the former farmer into pump failure. It was predictable as the seasonal rains in the South.

One spring day, Joe's doctor decided to admit him into the hospital for intravenous medication instead of the usual pill adjustments. Just a "two-day tune up," his doctor joked.

Well, two days in the hospital is no luxury resort vacation. On his final day in Joe spiked a 104 degree fever and his body vibrated like Jell-o from shaking chills. He had suffered a clot and infection in the arm vein with the intravenous line – a complication called thrombophlebitis. But this domino effect didn't end there. He was taken to the operating room to remove the vein out of fear the infection would not clear up, despite being started on a several week course of potent intravenous antibiotics. An innocent two-day tune-up turned into a several week ordeal.

Nursing Home Story

Dr. Joseph Ouslander, Senior Associate Dean for Geriatric Programs at Florida Atlantic University, describes a common scenario in a 2011 essay published in the *New England Journal of Medicine.* Similar situations occur daily in nursing homes and assisted living facilities across the United States:

A 90-year-old nursing home resident with Alzheimer's disease, advanced heart failure and chronic arthritis pain develops a dry cough and fever. The on-call doctor is paged and reflexively refers the unfamiliar frail senior to the emergency room. She is found to be stable in the ER and diagnosed with mild pneumonia. Her treatment: hospital admission for intravenous fluids and antibiotics. The next day she becomes confused, climbs out of her hospital bed and fractures her hip. One week later, she returns to the nursing home. Final cost: $10,000 and much pain, suffering and disability for a frail senior. Hip fractures in elders often serve as the key event leading to rapid decline, with high death rates by one year after the fracture.

Dr. Ouslander proposes an alternative way this 'script' could have played out: The night nurse evaluates the 90-year-old lady with cough and fever using a standardized process and phones an on-call nurse practitioner who knows the resident well. The nurse reports the stable vital signs and benign examination findings. No chest pain or trouble breathing. No swelling in the legs – a sign of heart failure. The nurse practitioner agrees the lady can be seen in the morning at which time an antibiotic and more fluids are ordered. The nurse practitioner diagnoses likely pneumonia and the lady's substitute decision-maker agrees that avoiding the hospital is best. A few days later the lady is much improved. The cost: $200 and no pain, suffering or added disability for a frail senior.

In fact, I propose that the antibiotic could have been initiated immediately, not the following day, to further reduce chances that frail lady would deteriorate and require hospitalization.

Untold Dangers of Hospitalization: Wilting While Under Care

Sit down while reading this chapter because you might get suddenly woozy when you learn about the dizzying list of risks and dangers that abound in hospitals. Isn't the hospital a nurturing, safe-zone for the sick? They do all sorts of tests to diagnose illness and have such nice nurses and qualified doctors, after all. That may be true, but it is not the whole story. There are many hidden risks lurking in hospital rooms and hallways: deadly infections that spread like wildfire; over-testing and radiation exposure; procedures that can cause complications including intravenous lines and bladder catheters; biopsies and surgeries based upon results of the myriad tests done; and too many medications and potent drugs with serious potential side effects. Incredibly, many hospital dangers wreak havoc on seniors even while the sudden illness that sent them there is improving! Older folks can quickly wilt while under care!

Daily Function Loss and Forced Dependence

Each hospital risk described below can contribute to a cycle of loss of function and independence from hospitalization. Loss of function and independence is the common thread that leads to loss of quality of life, dignity and life meaning. Loss of independence lands these frail folks into nursing homes or assisted living facilities. Bear in mind, it is not only the frail who are susceptible to hospital wilting risks. Any adult can be devastated by hospital-related complications.

Each stay in the hospital can chip away at an older adult's ability to perform daily living activities such as toileting, bathing, dressing, walking, and, of course, hobbies and interests. These deficits occur even when the illness that sent them to the hospital has been cured or is improving! The frail senior living independently or with some assistance gets by with a routine for making it to the bathroom in time, eating most meals prepared with just the right taste and consistency, and dressing independently even if a button or two is left undone. They can lose these abilities with the forced dependence of a hospital stay. While in the hospital, elders are commonly kept bedridden and unable to get to the bathroom, soon feeling humiliation at the loss of continence. Body muscles atrophy, transforming simple chores such as walking or standing up from a chair into improbable and unsafe tasks. Meals are placed out of reach on a sliding table; no matter, the food is cold and has all the wrong tastes, textures and consistencies to satisfy an aging, picky palate. Tubes and catheters magnify these function-loss concerns. The end result is a cycle of loss of function leading to loss of quality of life leading to loss of dignity as frail elders must be moved out of their own home into assisted living or a nursing home. This move is often done 'against their will' and leads to anger and ever more dependency on others for daily survival.

Bladder Catheters Gone Wild

It is hard to believe that between 20 and 50 percent of bladder catheters (Foley) are inserted unnecessarily and without clear rationale, according to published studies! Most of these needless procedures occur in emergency rooms, often without a doctor's order to do so. The elderly, it seems, are at greatest risk for avoidable urinary catheters and its potential complications. Urinary tract infections are responsible for more than one-third of hospital-related infections, with catheters causing the majority of these. What are the actual reasons for someone to appropriately get a short-term bladder catheter? First, if someone is unable to pee. A mechanical blockage such as enlarged prostate can cause inability to pee. When the urine suddenly gets trapped and cannot come out it causes a truly painful emergency that can damage the kidneys. A floppy (neurogenic) bladder can also lead to inability to pee, wherein the bladder muscles cannot contract and empty out the urine. This floppy bladder problem commonly complicates stroke, multiple sclerosis, Parkinson's disease and spinal cord injury. A second reason to insert a catheter is for close monitoring of the amount of urine output in critically ill people. Third, Foley catheters can help divert urine away from an advanced pressure ulcer. Fourth, it is for convenience and comfort in those who are terminally ill. Fifth, catheters may be needed after surgery for a short time.

In truth, catheters are anything but comfortable. These tubes cause embarrassment, loss of quality of life, inconvenience, difficulty getting around, and are a reminder to people they suffer from failing health. Catheters also tether people to the bed and make simple tasks more difficult. They can cause discomfort and pain. Complications include serious urinary tract infection and life-threatening sepsis. For additional tips on urinary infections and catheters, see the Red Flags section.

Tests, Procedures and Surgery

Tests, procedures and operations have their own inherent risks which should be explained to patients or caregivers when the doctor gets signed informed consent. Older folks, having limited reserves and less tolerability to body insults, are particularly vulnerable to complications. Seniors must consider long and hard whether the benefits of surgery or any procedure is worth the risks. Joan Rivers' tragic death, though it did not occur in the hospital setting, is a lesson to all of us that even simple procedures have great danger and unpredictability in older adults.

Malnutrition

Older folks have an uphill battle with adequate nutrition when they are hospitalized. First, they may have less appetite due to an illness that sent them into the hospital. Second, elders can have decreased ability to communicate and walk, making it hard to ask for and eat meals. Third, the meals are often cold and out of arm's reach. By the time the patient notices the tray after a soporific slumber, someone whisks it away untouched. Fourth, even hot meals can be tasteless to the elderly. Meals are usually disease-restricted such as low-salt or diabetic diet. No spices are added. Older folks typically lose smell and taste perception as they age, Disease-restricted diets combined with cold food with an unappealing texture is a recipe for bland and tasteless. What's more, elders may lose their ability to reach the tray and self-feed because of their acute sickness. The result of all this is loss of weight and muscle mass, as well as reduced strength and bone density. The final common pathway: loss of independence when an older adult can no longer do daily living tasks they did prior to the hospital trip. Most seniors never get back all that lost function.

Bed Rest: Loss of Muscle, Bone Density and Strength

Bed rest is worshipped in the ER and hospital. Yet it is perhaps the worst affliction for older folks. Many hospital workers reason incorrectly that keeping seniors in bed is best because they are safer there. There is less chance to fall. It also requires worker strain to lift infirm patients out of bed. Frail elders commonly feel weak or dizzy and might be having pain. Best not to bother them, hospital workers reason. Another common cause for bed rest is the senior who is tube-tied and tethered. Bladder catheters, intravenous lines, oxygen tubing, heart monitor wires, drainage tubes and feeding tubes may be inserted into older folks. These tethers can transform a hospital bed into a confining spider web.

Why is bed rest like a plague for older folks? We normally lose muscle mass as we age. Bed rest magnifies the problem. A 2007 *Journal of the American Medical Association* study found that healthy seniors with an average age of 67 years who were placed at bed rest for 10 days lost *two pounds* of muscle in the legs! Even young muscles at rest lose as much as 10 percent of their strength every two days. And unused muscles, tendons and ligaments tend to shrink, causing contractures and loss of joint function.

To make matters worse, rested bones lose their density and strength quickly, leading to greater risk of broken bones. Staying in bed can also cause the aging body's blood volume to shrink by about half a liter, thus making elders ever more prone to a cycle of dehydration, low blood pressure and falls. Finally, bed rest leads to loss of breathing stamina and thus limited function and exercise ability. Wow! It seems wise to quickly get off your butt and strut. It is also important to ask doctors and nurses daily if tubes and catheters are absolutely necessary or if they can be removed. Be sure to get all necessary equipment to make walking and sitting in a chair safe and possible.

Urine Incontinence

Up to half of hospitalized elderly folks have incontinence. Many seniors have this humiliating condition thrust upon them during their hospital stay when they cannot carry out their usual toileting routines or become less mobile than at home. Sedating medications and pain can also contribute, as do the web of catheters, heart monitor wires and others lines mentioned earlier.

Pressure Sores

Nasty and difficult to heal pressure ulcers can form within hours in older adults in an emergency room or hospital. Some key contributors are a hard stretcher, infrequent repositioning on a bed or stretcher, too much bed rest, inadequate protein in diet, reduced muscle and fat layer overlying bony protrusions where pressure is greatest, and over-sedation.

Falls

Falls in the elderly may be the first clue of a major change in health status, even if no significant injury occurs. Loss of muscle strength is a major contributing factor to falls. Weakened bone strength ups the risk for serious fractures. High hospital beds are a danger to a confused or determined senior who attempts to scale those heights in the dark of night. Sedating medication and overmedication remain common contributing factors for falls in the elderly. Incredibly, it is estimated that sixty percent of significant falls happen while seniors are *in* the hospital. Note, too, that older adults are 5 to 10 times more likely to die in the 3 months following hip fracture.

Nasty Hospital-Acquired Infections

The list of infections any person can catch inside the hospital is akin to an FBI Hundred Most Wanted list of crafty microscopic murderers. MRSA is likely most feared because that bug is resistant to most antibiotics, but bacteria such as Pseudomonas, Klebsiella, and vancomycin-resistant enterococcus (VRE) cause serious illnesses. Furthermore, these bugs might require treatment with two or three potent intravenous antibiotics and cure is not guaranteed. C. Diff is also widespread in hospitals and can cause severe intestinal disease in already sick folks. Furthermore, the number of cases of C. Diff diarrhea has doubled in the past decade with more cases caused by a resistant form of the disease.

Each year 700,000 hospital-caused infections are diagnosed in the United States, causing 75,000 deaths. How are hospital infections spread? Invasive devices lead to bacterial nests where the tube is connected to the body. The list of tube types includes bladder catheters, breathing tubes, intravenous catheters, drainage tubes and central line access to major veins. Invasive procedures and surgeries also pose risk for getting an infection. What's more, infections are easily spread from bacteria that live on surfaces of hospital furniture like beds or sliding tables, or medical equipment. C. Diff. spores, for instance, can survive on bed linens or rails, room fixtures or medical devices. What is concerning is studies have estimated that up to 38 percent of urinary catheter insertions are unnecessary and antibiotics are prescribed or continued unnecessarily up to 50 percent of the time!

Would it shock you to learn that a common mode of infection spread is off the hands of nurses, doctors, aides and visitors? Hand washing and stethoscope hygiene in hospitals is horrific. Surveys have shown that less than half of medical workers comply with hand hygiene recommendations. Patients and visitors do not fair any better in this regard. There has, in fact, been discussion in the medical literature about banning the handshake in healthcare settings. C. Diff diarrhea infection, for example, can be passed on with handshaking, and alcohol-based hand cleansers are ineffective against this tough bug. Perhaps there is good logic in the Japanese greeting that is simply a short bow. It is concerning that hand washing alone is not sufficient. A 2014 study published in *Mayo Clinic Proceedings* found that a doctor's stethoscope often carries more bacteria than their hands! Yet rarely do doctors clean their stethoscope between patients, if at all. Alcohol wipes and alcohol-based hand solutions are all effective at reducing contamination of stethoscope surfaces. Even neckties and clothing have been found to harbor and spread bacteria. Cleaning neckties and shirt sleeves with alcohol wipes, however, may not be such a good idea.

The key question remains: Will patients have the courage to tell their doctors, nurses and allied health workers to wash their hands, stethoscopes and other devices before examining them? Likely not and many patients are too ill to speak up. This is why placing a self-printed sign in a standing picture frame in plain view can help. See the 'Tips' section below for what your framed sign should say.

C. Difficile Diarrhea Epidemic: Shedding Light, Not Spores

This intestinal infection can cause severe diarrhea, vomiting, abdominal pain, fever or death. C. Diff, as it is nicknamed, has become an explosive epidemic and growing threat to older folks in hospitals, nursing homes and the community. This bacterium can live for weeks as impervious spores on contaminated surfaces, medical equipment and furniture. Bleach-based cleaners are necessary since typical hospital cleaners and soaps do not kill the spores. Surprisingly, recent research by the Centers for Disease Control and Prevention (CDC) found that only one-quarter of cases are contracted in the hospital. Most sufferers were already carriers of the bacteria and developed the illness after receiving antibiotics in the hospital. Spores are contracted by spread from feces to infected surfaces which then enter by swallowing it after spore contact with the mouth. That person then is a carrier of C. Diff and can develop active infection if conditions are ripe such as receiving antibiotic treatment. Why antibiotic treatment? Simply, the antibiotics kill good competing bacteria that normally live in the intestines, thus allowing C. Diff to flourish and release its toxins.

Sadly, research has found that as much as 50 percent of antibiotic use is unnecessary. In the community, common antibiotics such as levofloxacin, ciprofloxacin, cephalexin, ceftin and other cephalosporins are the most common precipitants of C. Diff infection because these potent drugs indiscriminately kill many types of bacteria, including the good intestinal bacteria. Risk factors for hospital-associated C. Diff infection include previous hospitalization, older age, antibiotic usage, suppressed immune system, nasogastric tubes, intestinal surgery and inflammatory bowel disease (ulcerative colitis, Crohn's disease). Stomach acid-lowering medications might also up risk by allowing safe passage of C. Diff through the normally acidic stomach into the intestines, and possibly altering normal bacterial growth in a less acidic environment.

Some Tips to Prevent C. Diff Spread:

- Identify C. Diff early as possible by the foul odor of stool caused by the chemical p-cresol. It is most contagious in its earliest stage. Interestingly, some dogs in the Netherlands have been trained to detect p-cresol and have a sense of smell 300-fold more sensitive to this chemical. Researchers in the Netherlands take the dogs on hospital rounds trying to halt infection spread.
- Once identified, wear gloves and gown, if possible. Wash all room surfaces with bleach daily. Hand washing with soap and water should last a minimum of 30 to 60 seconds. Get a medical evaluation and prompt treatment started as well.
- Question any antibiotic prescription for older adults. While these drugs may be reassuring, the CDC suggests up to half of antibiotics prescribed may be unnecessary. The worst offenders are related to ciprofloxacin, levofloxacin, cephalexin, and ceftin. C. Diff may not show itself for weeks after antibiotic treatment so a connection may not be made. Make no mistake: Antibiotics should be avoided or limited to lower doses and shorter courses of treatment whenever possible. Even in the hospital, ask the doctor if antibiotic treatment can be safely avoided or limited due to C. Diff concerns. They should understand the concern. After all, recurrence and treatment failure are commonly encountered with C. Diff.
- A recent analysis of twenty quality studies found that probiotics (Lactobacillus species and Saccharomyces boulardii) can be helpful in preventing antibiotic-associated diarrhea.
- Avoid stomach acid-lowering drugs such as ranitidine, famotidine, omeprazole, pantoprazole and all their chemical cousins when possible. Once again, ask the primary care provider if that medication is truly necessary or limit therapy to a few weeks.

Adverse Drug Reactions and Over-Prescribing of Medications

Medications can cure and medications can kill. Older adults are most vulnerable to drug side effects and bad reactions – known as adverse drug events – especially in the hospital setting. Patient harm due to medication reactions is cited as the second most common complication of being in the hospital. How common is it? Between 6 and 30 percent of those hospitalized will suffer harm from medication. And the elderly are at greatest risk because they have multiple chronic ailments, are already taking many medications, and an aging body is less able to process medications. It is not uncommon for seniors to be given drugs considered too risky for older adults.

While in an acute care hospital, prescribed medications pile up more quickly than dirty laundry in a basket. Potent intravenous antibiotics, stomach acid-lowering drugs, sleeping pills, blood thinners, higher doses of blood pressure medication, pain relievers, constipation medications, anti-nausea drugs, and on and on. Rarely are these medications stopped prior to discharge to a lower level of care facility or home. It is difficult for patients or families to distinguish what drugs are truly needed from those that can be avoided (see Medication Madness chapter).

Sensory Isolation

An older adult gets whisked by ambulance to the ER and winds up on a hospital unit without needed hearing aids, dentures, eyeglasses, magnifying glass, music players, books or other devices they rely upon. Sometimes these items are brought in but get lost during the hospital stay. This can contribute to sensory isolation when an older adult can barely hear, see or communicate with hospital staff. Discussions with doctors and nurses about their condition are barely audible or understood. Seniors may get few visitors during limited visitation times. In addition, they may be 'snowed under' by heavy duty medications used for pain, insomnia or confusion. At times it is overstimulation in the environment that discombobulates the elderly. Too-bright lights; people going in and out, back and forth; incessant poking, prodding, turning, awakening; and beeping monitors and squealing alarms. As with sensory isolation, overstimulation can also add up to acute confusion, diminished awareness of one's environment, and inability to maintain focus and attention – a dangerous condition known as delirium (see below).

Deadly, Deceptive Delirium

This serious disorder has taken on various cultural meanings. For instance, students often feel 'delirious' from studying all night for an exam. Another example: The Prince song titled, "I Get Delirious" in which singer Prince croons his lament about his inability to function or remain focused when he is around the woman he loves. Actually, delirium represents the body and mind's responses to generalized brain dysfunction caused by hundreds of possible conditions. Some common contributing factors include infection, blood chemistry abnormalities, underlying dementia, low oxygen level, sensory deprivation or overstimulation, dehydration, certain medications, and serious medical illnesses like stroke or sepsis. Studies have identified several key risk factors that spark delirium: Bladder catheters, physical restraints, malnutrition and use of three or more medications.

What does delirium look like? This brain fog disease can cause restlessness, confusion, and disorientation as illustrated by the thrashing patient who throws off covers and pulls out catheters or intravenous lines. A delirious patient might misperceive these lines and tubes to be snakes, for instance. Or delirium can resemble the quiet, drowsy senior who sleeps much of the day, but may show lucidity, agitation or confusion at times. This low activity version of delirium can resemble depression. Either way, those who develop delirium during a hospital stay have been found to have between 22 and 75 percent mortality rate. They are also at high risk of death in the months that follow a hospitalization. Those diagnosed with delirium when first admitted into the hospital have death rates as high as 1 in 4. Sadly, delirium is frequently missed by doctors caring for the elderly and written off as dementia or depression. One study found nearly one-third of elderly emergency room patients suffering from delirium were sent home!

Why are Elderly Folks Sent to the Emergency Room unnecessarily?

- Panic by loved ones who are solely responsible for care when a senior suffers a fall or feels suddenly ill
- Lack of advance plan to promptly arrange to see a doctor or nurse practitioner for urgent medical illness. It can be hard to find a medical practice that will see sick older folks urgently before sending them to the ER.
- Delay in identifying illness that is brewing over a few days. Older adults often have gradual deterioration in their condition with vague signs of sickness until their illness reaches crisis levels.
- Primary care doctors are frequently too busy to fit complicated older patients into office hours so they reflexively refer them to the ER.
- Family members insist on sending loved ones to the emergency room. They mistakenly believe the ER and hospital are always the safest place to be for their ill loved one who lives at a nursing home or assisted living. For life-threatening illness, that may be true although a frail older adult in the last couple years of their life often cannot benefit much from aggressive hospital treatments. Palliative care planning is sometimes the wisest choice.

Why are Elderly Folks Admitted into the Hospital Unnecessarily?

1. **Lazy Admission-** Old folks often have many complex medical ailments. So when a primary care or covering doctor gets called about a sick elderly patient, it is easier to send that patient to the ER and have them admitted into the hospital until the complexities get sorted out – even if the illness turns out to be a mild pneumonia or simple urinary tract infection. Sometimes the ER doctor wants to rush an older patient through the system but fears missing a diagnosis in a frail person they are unfamiliar with. To minimize liability of missing something, the ER doctor errs on the "safe" side (safe for doctor, not patient) and saves time dealing with difficult

medical and social issues by admitting the patient into the hospital and rushing them up to a bed on a medical ward.

2. **Unscrupulous Admission** – Several large hospital chains across the United States had been under investigation by the Justice Department for alleged practices to increase admissions of older folks to generate higher revenue, even if that patient could have been sent home! Consider the following excerpt from a 2014 *New York Times* article by journalists Julie Creswell and Reed Abelson:

   Every day the scorecards went up, where they could be seen by all of the hospital's emergency room doctors. Physicians hitting the target to admit at least half of the patients over 65 years old who entered the emergency department were color-coded green. The names of doctors who were close were yellow. Failing physicians were red.

   A scary thought, to be sure, that emergency room doctors' jobs were alleged to be on the line if they did not bring in as many elderly folks as possible into the dangerous hospital environment.

3. **Malpractice Fears** – Doctors practice defensive medicine out of fear of lawsuits. It is harder to be sued successfully if a doctor admits a frail older adult into the hospital rather than trying to do what is best for that patient by keeping them out. If the patient does poorly outside the hospital, the doctor can easily be blamed for lackadaisical care. If the patient does poorly because of hospital complications... well, that's just the risks of receiving modern medical care. It is not just the doctors who have liability fear. Nursing homes, assisted living facilities, and group homes are reluctant to provide more intensive illness management for moderately serious ailments and risk something going awry on their watch.

4. **Distorted Dollar Incentives** – Skilled nursing homes can get paid a much higher reimbursement rate to care for a senior just released from the hospital, as opposed to that person getting more intensive treatment in the same nursing home only, that is still classified as "routine" care. Assisted living facilities and group homes do not necessarily get paid any extra money for undertaking the greater risk and necessary care responsibilities for a sick elderly

resident getting hospital-level treatments like intravenous fluids and antibiotics.

5. **Lack of Care Goals Plan** – Each older adult should have in writing their care goals and wishes based upon their spiritual and religious beliefs, the seriousness of their medical conditions, and personal goals for the final stage of life. Do everything to prolong life? Do not resuscitate? No hospitalization? Hospitalization and simple treatments okay but no invasive tests or treatments? Comfort care only? Each individual must choose what is right for them (see Don't Worry, Die Happy chapter for more details).
6. **No Medical Care at Home** – Lack of planning to get 'hospital at home' care arranged promptly in cooperation with your primary care doctor. This approach to care cuts out the middleman (hospital) to bring certain hospital-level treatments to the senior in a safer, familiar environment for less serious illnesses. This approach has been safe and successful with greater patient satisfaction when used in countries across the globe. In the United States, it can be difficult to coordinate between doctor, home health or infusion nurses and caregivers in a timely fashion. Payment obstacles exist for some of these services provided in a home setting.

Wise Tips When Hospital Admission is Required

Doctors must get signed informed consent from patients before doing any procedure or operation, explaining key risks versus benefits. Dr Muriel Gillick has asked this common sense question: Why is not the same informed consent standard expected before a doctor sends an older adult to an emergency room or hospital, wherein dangers are rampant and risks run high? Dr. Gillick, Clinical Professor at Harvard Medical School, wrote the following astute comment in an essay on frail elderly going to the hospital for care:

When physicians recommend hospitalization for treatment of acute illness without offering alternatives, they imply and patients assume that it is the only safe and effective choice.

Tips for the Necessary Hospital Stay

Be proactive when an older adult must stay in the hospital. Try to make the stay as much like being at home as possible. But do not count on hospital staff alone to fulfill all of grandma's needs, nor to minimize all potential hospital harms. Most hospital staff are devoted and do a fine job, but they have limited time for each patient. Family, friends and volunteers must pick up the slack and serve as surrogate nursing assistant and patient advocate.

- **Bedside Guard**: A friend, relative, volunteer or paid caregiver should ideally be at an older adult's bedside all day, although night shift might be most important when hospital staffing is thinner and elderly patients are more likely to become confused and get hurt in the dark of night.
- **Feeding Grandma**: Do not depend on hospital food alone for grandma or grandpa to get adequate nutrition – assuming he or she is allowed to take food by mouth. First, consider eating limitations such as no dentures available or difficulty swallowing. What is the soonest grandma will be allowed to try eating? Second, urge doctors to eliminate restrictive diets in frail older adults such as low-salt or low-fat diets. Third, supply foods with appealing textures, scents, spices, flavors, sweets and favorite foods when possible. Consider bringing food in from home or a preferred restaurant. Cardboard-bland won't get grandma's parched palate purring or intestinal motor running. Fourth, determine how much help grandma will need with actual eating while hospitalized. She might need to be encouraged and fed for a while. An occasional chocolate indulgence, milkshake, or other favorite treat after a meal can be both meaningful and helpful.
- **Serene, Just-Like-Home Surroundings**: Avoid Sensory Isolation. Make that hopefully short hospital stay feel as much like home as possible. Transform that bland, disorienting hospital room and make it come alive: display a few favorite photos of loved ones; bring brightly-colored flowers (as allowed); provide pleasant and pleasing scents such as lavender, citrus or mint (as allowed); play soothing music on a simple CD player or find a music channel on the television; allow bright light in during daytime by opening

curtains and exposing pleasant outside views; avoid overstimulation and keep low level lighting during evening hours; provide hearing aids, amplifier, dentures, eyeglasses, magnifying glass or other needed devices so grandma can keep in touch with her surroundings; orient grandma with a large calendar and clock; maintain regular social contact throughout the day by spreading out times for visitors rather than everybody storming in at once to say hello.

- **Keep Grandma Moving**: Ask the physical therapist for advice on what exercises and activities grandma can safely do immediately. Discuss with doctors everyday when tethers like catheters or intravenous lines or monitor wires can be removed for better mobility and less risk of complications. Loved ones can also have grandma do simple arm and leg lifts using light wrist or ankle velcro weight sets. These repetitions can be done in bed or a chair to keep the muscles moving and blood pumping. Get grandma out of bed to a chair several times daily as soon as allowed. Other activities to do in the chair: deep breathing and sucking on an incentive spirometer gadget to expand the lungs, resistance band pulls, and leg and arm range of motion bending and straightening to prevent contractures and joint tightening. Do not depend only on a 30-minute physical therapy visit once a day during the hospitalization. Note: the key is to focus on maintaining function and independence physically, as well as meaning and will to live spiritually and mentally.
- **Try Clearing the Drug Fog**: Discuss cutting back on some meds as discharge approaches such as PPI for stomach acid, sedatives, sleeping pills or behavior meds.
- **Help Prevent Falls**: Not so simple. Keep the hospital bed low to ground. Pay attention to diet, exercise, sensory stimulation and medication advice as discussed in this section. It is also advisable to have friends or loved ones there to assist grandma as much as possible to help avoid slips and falls.
- **Infection Control**: Take note if doctors and nurses are washing hands before and after contact with you. Do they wear gloves, gowns and masks as needed? Discomfort aside, it is not unreasonable to

ask medical personnel to wipe clean their stethoscopes or other equipment with rubbing alcohol or alcohol-based hand sanitizer. These disinfectants are proven and effective approaches to reducing infection spread. Consider simply printing out a sign and placing it in a standing frame on the sliding table near grandma. It should contain the following message: "*Please wash hands and sanitize stethoscopes and other medical equipment before your examination or procedure.*" An alternative sign with some humor: "*Serious Allergy: Grandpa is highly allergic to MRSA, Pseudomonas and C. Diff. Please wash hands and sanitize stethoscopes and other devices as you care for grandpa.*"

- **Get Grandma Home**: Get seniors out of the hospital quickly as possible and arrange for plenty of doctor, nurse and caregiver support at home based upon qualifying ailments.

Avoiding Needless Admissions

Once the emergency room doctor or hospital-based doctor (hospitalist) suggests a hospital stay is likely, ask what will be done in the hospital that cannot be done at a sub-acute care facility like rehab or at the house, assisted living or nursing home that grandma considers as her home. Also inquire about getting medical care at home services – known as 'hospital at home' – or simply hospice or home health assistance outside the hospital setting. These are potential alternatives to hospitalization that are too often dismissed by the medical community, but might well be appropriate particularly for frail seniors. In fact, treatment can be initiated in the emergency room and additional treatments continued as 'medical care at home' over the next few days. But you must suggest this approach to avoid an inpatient hospital stay or it is not likely to be offered.

Alternatively, have the ER doctor call a trusted primary care doctor to discuss if admission into the hospital is truly needed.

Let the ER doctor know about grandma's wishes for limited treatments in which case the usual automatic admission process might be changed even by doctors who tend to be more aggressive with admitting older folks. Provide any needed documentation for medical directives and wishes.

The surest way to avoid hospital admission: do not call the ambulance in the first place! Instead, call a home visiting doctor, nurse practitioner, or hospice and palliative care nurse for comfort care. Note that grandma might fear she will never return home again or will die if she is taken to an emergency room. The fear is not unrealistic.

Alternatives to Hospitalization

Considering all the dangers of a stay in the hospital, it may not be surprising that 20 to 25 percent of seniors released from the hospital are readmitted to a hospital within 30 days! Perhaps it is just *being in the hospital* that makes the elderly sick enough to again require hospitalization for a different problem? Dangerous hospital-acquired infections. Malnutrition and loss of appetite. Loss of muscle mass and strength. Forced bed rest and dependence. Loss of functional abilities. Overmedication. Disorientation, confusion and social and sensory deprivation. Complications from invasive procedures. Wow! Even if the acute medical illness that sent the person into the ER and hospital has been successfully treated, the complication list above is long and intimidating and can surely lead to new problems that result in repeat hospitalization.

Dr. Gillick has said in private correspondence with this author (JC), "I think lots of people would like to live longer but are more concerned about maintaining their level of function and their comfort." Each person must formulate the plan that fits his or her personal needs. As one approaches the last phase of life, if a person values comfort, quality of life, and functional independence more than simply the extension of life at all cost, then one might consider a "hospital at home" approach to care. That is, bringing needed basic treatments such as intravenous fluids and antibiotics to the patient in the home setting. Dr. Gillick prefers to call this "medical care at home" as she correctly points out that this care is *not* the same as hospital-based care. Care cannot be as aggressive. Monitoring will not be as reliable and extensive, but the benefit is fewer dangers than being in a hospital. In addition, there is the best possible advantage: all the comforts of home. Those who choose this approach get to sleep in their own bed, have the company of friends and loved ones all day, pass the time doing the leisure activities they usually enjoy, eat foods they typically like, and get the care and attention not possible in a busy hospital setting. When choosing an assisted living, group home or nursing home you might want to consider how much treatment they are willing to perform at the facility. Will they allow intravenous infusions to perhaps prevent a hospital stay?

There are, of course, limits to what ailments can be treated with medical care at home. At some point it may be wise to consider a palliative care or hospice approach for those in the last stage of life. This means relinquishing most invasive interventions and focusing on simple treatments and comfort care.

It is not unusual for medics to come and evaluate an older adult who is sick or has fallen. Medics can help the senior off the floor, give simple assistance, and do a basic evaluation. They will usually abide by your wishes to avoid hospital transport if comfort care is the goal or the illness episode seems to have improved. At worst, they will ask you to sign a refusal to get transported to the hospital.

Urgent care facilities are not an ideal option for frail elderly. These freestanding centers can, however, be convenient for healthier seniors with minor issues like a small laceration, twisted ankle, or respiratory infection, for instance.

Useful Websites to Help Research Hospital Quality and Rankings

http://www.medicare.gov/hospitalcompare/search.html

http://health.usnews.com/best-hospitals/area

http://www.consumerreports.org/health/doctors-hospitals/hospital-ratings.htm

(Subscription required for Consumer Reports Site)

http://www.hospitalsafetyscore.org/

http://health.usnews.com/best-hospitals/rankings/cardiology-and-heart-surgery

http://www.sts.org/quality-research-patient-safety/sts-public-reporting-online

http://www.beckershospitalreview.com/lists/100-hospitals-and-health-systems-with-great-heart-programs-2014.html

Also, search your state health department for heart procedure rankings and hospital safety information.

DANGER 7. MALPRACTICE FEARS AND DEFENSIVE MEDICINE

Malpractice lawsuits are to doctors what Kryptonite is to Superman. It weakens them and disrupts their very core. Hospitals fear medical malpractice as well and they have far deeper pockets. A publicized lawsuit can have devastating consequences on the hospital's reputation— and bottom line. Why should a patient really care much about physicians' high malpractice insurance costs or a hospital's lawsuit anxiety? If lost sleep for doctors and hospital CEOs was the only consequence then folks should not much care. Lawsuit fears, however, have been transformed into defensive medical practice which *does* have direct and grave consequences for you, the patient.

In the American medico-legal system, doing too much is far safer than doing too little. Hardly a conversation passes among physicians, nurses or other healthcare workers without the poetic phrase, "cover your butt" or "CYA" being mentioned.

What exactly is defensive medicine? This overly-cautious approach to medical care comes in the form of ordering unnecessary tests, treatments or hospitalizations with the hope of shielding doctors from a lawsuit. It places doctor fears above care that best serves a patient's interests. Defensive medicine also exists in the form of *lack* of needed care for complex diseases and high-risk patients. Once considered just an American medicine problem, defensive medicine concerns have grown more prominent in other countries such as China, Japan, Italy, Israel and the United Kingdom, based upon medical journal reports. Consider the following actual examples of blatant defensive medical care:

A middle-aged woman arrives at an emergency room complaining of chest pains. Her breathing is okay and she reports no other concerning symptoms. In fact, she underwent a stress test last year when she experienced similar symptoms. The test was normal then. The doctor in training reviewed her prior records, discussed the situation with her family doctor, and they concluded she is low-risk for a serious heart problem. As the young doctor prepared to discharge the lady, the ER doctor in charge insisted the woman be admitted into the hospital for overnight observation and undergo a nuclear stress test, imaging with significant radiation exposure.

"She may not need it, but treadmill stress tests like the one she had last year aren't always accurate, and being wrong is not worth the risk of getting sued," the charge doctor insisted, as reported in a 2013 issue of *Journal of the American Medical Association Internal Medicine*. The woman was sent home the following day after her nuclear stress test proved to be normal, as expected.

The following excerpt from Cal Woodward's essay printed in a 2010 issue of the *Canadian Medical Association Journal* sheds light on over-testing inherent in defensive medical practice. At some point in time, too much testing with dubious benefit for patients becomes the gold standard of care to which all doctors will be held accountable:

The 48-year-old man who came in for his routine check-up seemed the picture of health: fit guy, loves basketball, no sickly past. Yet his doctors performed a battery of tests that raised eyebrows in United States medical circles.

The patient had a colonoscopy normally done for older men, a calcium-deposit heart scan usually reserved for higher-risk patients and a prostate cancer screening test no longer routinely recommended...

Call it defensive medicine from the top down. The patient was President Barack Obama, who recently overhauled the American health care system but left one problem area untouched: the impulse to go overboard with expensive and invasive procedures of questionable benefit.

...Obama's doctors set an unexpectedly controversial example in his physical (exam) and, in some minds, conceivably imperiled his future health with excess radiation.

The first two cases above are examples of risky over-testing in both the emergency room and outpatient settings. In the emergency room, it is for "CYA" reasons; with the President, it happened because of a dubious belief that a normal result on random testing of all types means all is okay. In fact, tests are fallible. These tests also exposed the president to dangerous, and perhaps unnecessary, radiation that increases future cancer risk. The next true anecdote illustrates lawsuit fear run amuck:

An internist was called to the emergency room to evaluate a young man who arrived with chest pain. No illegal drugs were involved. The ER doctor concluded he was low-risk for true heart disease despite some minor irregularities on the young man's electrocardiogram which might have been due to his thin frame. The consulting internist looked at the top of the computerized electrocardiogram that included an automated interpretation: "Nonspecific repolarization abnormality, cannot exclude myocardial infarction." These canned computer readings are typically inaccurate and largely ignored. The test must be interpreted in proper context, like a thin chest wall which could mimic the noted changes.

Without much hesitation, the internist turned to his colleague, scratched his head and said, "I want to admit the patient into the intensive care unit."

The puzzled ER doctor asked for an explanation. The internist offered one: "How can I *not* send him to intensive care with 'Cannot exclude myocardial infarction' written all over his EKG?"

In the unlikely event the man did experience a true heart problem, the internist feared a lawsuit because the EKG machine "knew" the diagnosis and he ignored it. Sadly, his fears were not unrealistic as lawyers could make a doctor look foolish for ignoring an "obvious" diagnosis that even a machine knew. Diagnosing heart disease can be tricky.

Approximately 6 million chest pain sufferers visit American emergency rooms each year, with about 80 percent of them deemed to be at low risk for a heart problem. A defensive medicine approach like this case could inundate our intensive care and heart monitoring units, making them unavailable for true heart attack sufferers.

The following case illustrates the most subtle danger of defensive medicine – the absence of care availability in Chester County, Pennsylvania.

Exorbitant malpractice premiums and astronomical lawsuit settlements in Pennsylvania have, in the past, caused some neurosurgeons to close up shop and move to more favorable states. Many other brain surgeons have responded by simply avoiding high-risk surgeries like head trauma, brain bleeds and tumors, leaving seriously ill folks without prompt specialist care. These sick people have required transfer to nearby Lancaster County, resulting in the death of two patients during the one-hour ambulance ride, according to reports. As for neurosurgeons who continue to practice, a national survey found nearly three-quarters of brain surgeons admitted to ordering unnecessary imaging tests solely to reduce their malpractice liability risk. Another unintended consequence: This practice of over-testing can creep into the daily habits of all doctors and become the new standard of care. If a doctor does not order the million-dollar workup then patients (and lawyers) scowl at them with distrust.

Other examples of subtly absent or unavailable care because of malpractice mania include when surgeons, for instance, refuse to accept a patient who suffered botched or unsuccessful back surgery, not wanting to be a lawsuit target in case the outcome remains poor. Many surgeons will not operate to repair a problem in a patient who had recent surgery elsewhere, forcing that person to return to the surgeon who did the initial *unsuccessful* procedure. Also, fewer specialists nationwide are willing to be on call for emergency room patients since receiving payment is iffy, but high liability concern is ever present.

It is concerning from a defensive medicine standpoint that hospitals create protocols called "standardized procedures." These protocols can lead to unnecessary cost and pain for patients. An auto crash trauma patient, for example, may be subjected to a total-body CT scan that includes the head, neck, chest, abdomen and possibly a limb! It is not uncommon for these patients to be at low risk for serious injury. The costs can add up to tens of thousands of dollars; the massive radiation dose can pose a significant cancer risk as well. It is not uncommon for hospitals to develop new protocols in response to a lawsuit. These processes are developed with the hope of preventing a similar negative event. The certain result: Thousands of people may needlessly be subjected to new risks, pain, suffering and high costs for fear of that one rare event. It may be cheaper to create a protocol than to continuously educate staff to practice quality medical care. Consider this example:

A middle-aged woman is involved in an auto accident. She is brought in by ambulance to a nearby trauma center emergency room. She has a gash on her forehead, a bruised right arm, and no other concerns. The nurse inserts a catheter into to her bladder while she is left stark naked in the ER trauma room. Passing the tube is painful, and she is embarrassed as a few male hospital workers look on. She complains about the lack of privacy and the invasive procedures but is told, "Protocol requires all patients brought in as a trauma alert to receive a catheter." The next day, after she was sent home, the accident victim develops a bladder infection from insertion of the catheter. She is prescribed an antibiotic and then experiences an allergic reaction with red itchy blotches all over her skin. All this drama happened because of a relatively minor car accident. Mary did not know she had the right to refuse the bladder catheter or any test or treatment she felt was not needed. The hospital is required by law to respect her wishes, including refusal of treatment.

Emergency Room and Hospital Defensive Strategies to Avoid Getting Sued

1. **Emergency Care by Protocol:** Creating canned approaches to care for everybody can be harmful to many folks while helping just a few. An example is the woman's case above who was needlessly subjected to loss of dignity and pain and complications from an unnecessary bladder catheter.

2. **Ordering Unnecessary Imaging Tests or Labs:** Many published doctor surveys have found large majorities of doctors admit to ordering unnecessary tests, treatments and hospital admissions solely to reduce risk of getting sued – risks and discomfort for patients be damned. Frankly, the minority of doctors in those surveys were probably too embarrassed to admit they too practice defensive medicine. High-dose radiation exposure and reactions to contrast dye are real dangers from this practice. Moreover, over-testing can lead to riskier procedures when shadows or normal body variations on imaging are labeled "abnormalities" that must be further evaluated with biopsies or surgery.

3. **Calling in Unnecessary Consultants:** ER physicians commonly call for a specialist consultation simply to protect themselves from a lawsuit:

Example: 77 year-old Millie felt dizzy after a full day at the county fair. The temperature hovered in the upper 90's, and Millie did not drink much water during the day. Her daughter was worried and took her to the emergency room. Although it seemed clear her low blood pressure was caused by dehydration in combination with her blood pressure medication, the ER doctor called in a neurologist consultation. Why? With the remote chance Millie's symptoms were caused by a stroke, the neurologist would be responsible for the missed diagnosis, not the ER doctor.

4. **Avoidable Hospital Admissions:** Some ER physicians may not have the confidence to send you home with a self-limiting illness that will improve within a day or two. In essence, they fear a potential lawsuit if things deteriorate at home so they admit you for observation. In some cases, doctors may feel pressured to admit you into the hospital when you can be cared for at home. There have been well-publicized reports of some hospital systems pressuring doctors to order avoidable tests, procedures and hospitalizations simply to generate more income. Typical examples of hospital admissions that could have been managed at home include walking pneumonia, low-risk chest pain when a heart attack has been excluded with appropriate testing, and moderate dehydration. What is so bad about spending a night or two in the medical Marriott or healthcare Hilton? Some TLC and rest and relaxation could be much needed. Well, there are serious risks (see Risks of Hospitalization chapter). Anybody can contract serious infections or serious complications from tubes and catheters commonly used.

The corollary to unnecessary admissions, of course, is its polar opposite: when an overworked doctor who spends just a couple minutes with you wants to quickly order a test or two and then insists on sending you home. If you are feeling as bad or worse than when you arrived, especially if feeling seriously ill, you should refuse discharge and insist you cannot go home in that condition. This practice of rushing patients out the door to empty out the chaotic ER can prove quite dangerous.

A Few Key Points on Preventing Harms of Defensive Medicine and Malpractice Fears

- Defensive medicine builds a wall of suspicion between doctor and patient, severely damaging the once-revered doctor-patient relationship. Most patients will never know why a doctor seems aloof, abrupt, and suspicious of them. Defensive medical practice and fear of lawsuits might play a significant role.
- It has been argued that the high rate of survey reports that doctors *do* practice defensive medicine may not capture the true extent of defensive medicine. Doctors may convince themselves they did a great job by confirming no brain damage on a CT scan, for instance, while exposing a person to significant radiation risk. Any clinically competent physician knows most of the time when it is safe to send home a patient who suffered minor head injury, without doing costly and risky brain imaging. A relatively mild mode of injury (bumping an open kitchen cabinet versus a serious injury like a baseball bat smashing your head), a normal examination, a few hours of observation, and head injury precaution instructions to monitor for changes in condition over the next day or two will usually suffice. In fact, defensive medical practice can become an unconscious habit that makes doctors believe they are thorough.
- A thorough doctor can be reassuring when they report to you normal results on the million-dollar workup. As people must increasingly pay a share of the costs for care, however, excessive testing, treating and spending can financially devastate people. They might be on the hook to pay thousands of dollars in testing, treatment, hospitalization and physician consultation costs that may have been avoidable. Remember: It is your right as patient to question the necessity of advanced and risky tests or treatments. You can politely refuse them and reassure emergency workers you will get close follow up with your family doctor if symptoms persist. Watchful waiting for a day or two can, at times, be wise when illness is improving or is unlikely to be life-threatening.
- Ask the ER doctor directly what the cost of a procedure or lab test or x-ray is likely to cost, and what cheaper and safer alternatives

exist. Some primary care doctors do this routinely, but in the rushed environment of the emergency room you will have to be forceful in expressing your need to know upfront what costs will be (see also, ER Overcharges chapter).

- Let your doctors know upfront you are not interested in "just-in-case" tests or treatments. You want only what is quality, safe, patient-centered care. If a test or treatment seems optional and not vital for diagnosis and treatment, then politely refuse and let the doctors document in your record you refused that recommendation.
- Do not insist upon or demand specific tests because your neighbor or brother once had it done. As the saying goes: Be wary of what you ask, for you may get it! And it may not be what you really need. Another bad patient habit: Never threaten to sue people in the ER if things are not going your way. Emergency room staff will reflexively isolate and avoid you, or do every unnecessary test possible to reduce liability. Doctors need some reassurance they will be allowed to use clinical judgment and can practice in a comfort zone, without an axe swinging overhead. Ask for second opinions, help and reassurance from nurses and doctors if you question the quality of care you get.
- If the emergency room doctor wants to call in a specialist to evaluate you, ask politely if that specialist consult is truly necessary right now. How will the specialist change the diagnosis and treatment plan at that moment? Perhaps you can follow up with that specialist in the office when he or she is more awake? Ask nurses and doctors in the ER if they would use that specialist for their own family? That will tell you all you need to know about the confidence they have in that doctor. Is that consultant part of your health insurance network or will you be responsible for much of the doctor's bill? Even in-network specialist consults can add to your out-of-pocket costs. Of course, beware that specialists, as a rule, tend to order more fancy diagnostic tests or procedures.
- Do not confuse over-testing and over-treating with quality medical care. For life-threatening illness, erring on the side of over-testing

may be reasonable. Not true for common variety illnesses. Ask for the least risky tests or treatments first. As testing in the form of defensive medicine increases, excessive care can become the norm – the new standard of care. Many patients may then mistakenly feel cheated if *not* subjected to a risky and unnecessary million-dollar workup.

- What should you do for hospital admissions? Ask straight up if the admission is really necessary or can you get close attention or home healthcare treatment and monitoring services at your home. Consider asking the physician in charge for another opinion if the doctor treating you does not instill confidence or does not have logical explanations to justify your admission. You can ask the ER doctor to call your family doctor to determine if they can send you home with close follow up. If, on the other hand, the doctors believe your illness is high-risk and possibly life threatening, then stay the night!

DANGER 8. TRUE INFORMED CONSENT FOR PATIENTS: ELUSIVE OR ACHIEVABLE?

Let us be realistic. Can patients truly get informed consent in the age of blink-of-an-eye office visits? Ever more complex medical care makes even a doctor's head spin. There has recently been much chatter about "high-value care" with expectations of patient-centered medical decisions, reduction of unnecessary tests and treatments, and control of costs. It is hard to take this chatter seriously. As long as doctor visits are fleeting; as long as time-pressured physicians reflexively send sick people to emergency rooms before evaluating them; as long as malpractice fears reign and lead to defensive medical practice; as long as primary care doctor visit compensation remains relatively low compared to pay for performing procedures, rendering it not worth the trouble to squeeze sick patients into an overly-hectic schedule; as long as medical care trends favor hi-tech and low-compassion; as long as techno-tests, treatments and procedures overshadow hand-holding and basic patient education, then true informed consent will remain an elusive phantom holed up in the crypts of medical care. It is my fear, sadly, that actual informed consent does not exist in most patient encounters.

What exactly *is* informed consent? Most people (including many doctors) believe this process is defined and satisfied by a patient signing a one-page standard consent form before undergoing a risky test, treatment or procedure. The consent form is, in fact, the *final* legal step in the whole consent process – the proof an interaction of some kind took place. The process of informed consent involves explanations of risks and benefits and alternatives for a test, treatment or procedure. Brochures, models or video aids might be part of the educational process. Informed consent should also allow time for patients to let the information stew, discuss it with loved ones, and then ask the doctor additional questions. How many people actually research, contemplate and analyze information then ask astute and detailed questions before undergoing a non-emergency test or procedure? Any hands? What is worse, the process of informed consent, as weak as it may be nowadays, is reserved mostly for high-risk tests, treatments and surgeries. Yet, drug prescriptions are potentially high risk. No consent form is needed when a doctor hands a patient a prescription for potentially risky medication. What about informed consent for high levels of radiation exposure from imaging tests? Simply signing that consent form is not true or adequate informed consent (see also, Too Much Trust in Tests chapter).

How can we change the system and include actual informed consent for medication prescriptions? For referral to an emergency room or admission into a hospital as well? Surely these are also high-risk situations that warrant in-depth explanations of risks, benefits and alternatives. The answer to changing the inadequate status quo: "Patient-Power," of course! Learn what to ask in this book and then *demand* concise and full explanations of risks, benefits and other options in easily understood language and with time to digest all the facts. Then do some additional research on your own before reaching a final decision to accept or reject your doctor's recommendation. Sometimes doing *nothing* is the best care decision. Furthermore, a second opinion for major procedures or surgeries should be the golden rule.

Consider the following four fictional medication scenarios. Which pill would you be willing to take and which drug are you unlikely to use?

1. People who take this pill daily over the next eight years will have a 50 percent lower risk of suffering a stroke.
2. Among people who take this pill for eight years, there will be a two percent lower risk of suffering a stroke.
3. Among the 50 people who take this pill daily over the next eight years, one person will be spared a stroke
4. Between 96 and 98 percent of people will NOT suffer a stroke regardless of whether or not they take this medication daily for eight years. Of 100 people who *do take* this pill, 98 will NOT suffer a stroke and two people will suffer a stroke over the next eight years; without taking the pill, 96 people will NOT suffer a stroke and about four people will suffer a stroke.

How doctors frame or explain benefits against risks means everything. Actually, the four scenarios above are different ways of describing risk for the *same* medication. Turn off the television or music while reading the explanation that follows. It will require total concentration to absorb these explanations – something most people lack, by the way, when faced with prospects for major surgery or serious illness.

The 50 percent lower risk is a *relative* risk reduction that compares just pill takers versus pill avoiders who *do* suffer a stroke (small minority of people in the study). The two percent lower risk is an *absolute* risk, reminding us that the true overall stroke risk is quite small whether or not that medication is taken (96 to 98 percent of people will *not* suffer stroke either way). The final scenario explains risk in actual numbers, showing that whether or not you take that medication daily for eight years, your chances are great that you will NOT suffer a stroke (between 96 and 98 percent). If I had a 96 to 98 percent chance for anything, I would feel pretty good about things.

Unfortunately, clinical researchers and drug marketers frequently report and frame study results to doctors and patients similar to the first, most optimistic scenario. A 50 percent risk reduction sounds great! It is a no-brainer. I want that treatment or procedure! In actuality, your risk for that disease might be quite small whether or not you accept that proposed treatment. Many busy doctors do not have time to analyze the statistics of the latest study for drug therapy or more specialized treatments. Several surveys, in fact, have shown that when doctors were tested on statistical interpretations like the scenarios above, they failed miserably in interpreting results. Doctors usually overestimate actual benefits, meaning they succumb to commonly-used marketing bias. How, then, can doctors properly explain accurate risks versus benefits to patients when recommending a drug or procedure? Are these treatment recommendations hopelessly biased by sales and marketing slants? Are doctors uninformed about actual and subtle benefits and risks of a treatment? Can their recommendations be influenced by their own best interests rather than the patients' interests? Sadly, the answer to these questions is not uncommonly, "Yes."

Drug salespeople, in fact, usually report to doctors the positively-framed statistics about drug benefits. "You can offer your patients a 50 percent reduction in stroke risk if they take this drug," would be their hypothetical pitch, based upon how marketing departments frame clinical study results. Not surprisingly, side effect concerns are minimized. For instance, several major studies of drugs to lower cholesterol levels did not report frequency of major side effects. In fact, the Heart Protection Study had more than one-third of participants drop out from the study after taking simvastatin for about one month. These dropouts were never included in the results of the study even though many withdrew because of side effects. Cost may also be ignored, as may be reduced quality of life from adverse reactions or unintended consequences from that treatment.

Balloon Angioplasty: Poster Child for Pitfalls in Informed Consent

Balloon angioplasty is a procedure in which a wire is threaded into a leg or arm artery up to the heart. An inflatable balloon scrapes open a clogged heart-feeding artery. It is now well established that this procedure, which ends with insertion of a stent to prop the artery open, can save lives during a heart attack. What is also known is that a person suffering *mild angina* symptoms will derive little benefit from this invasive and risky procedure. In fact, several studies have found that optimal medication therapy, quitting smoking, and proper diet and exercise get better results than angioplasty for mild and *stable* heart disease. There is no reduction in heart attack or death risk with stent insertion for those who suffer from *stable* heart disease (as opposed to impending or actual heart attack).

It is shocking to hear the rationale cardiologists might use for performing these invasive angioplasty procedures to prop open a blocked artery. One study used focus group discussions with cardiologists to shed light on this issue. "The blockage is there so it is hard to ignore" is one reason put forth, despite knowing the procedure does not help stable patients, according to the best evidence. Some cardiologists may promote the procedure based upon an isolated past emotional experience when one patient died suddenly after they did *not* perform the procedure. This personal experience of patient death may have been unpredictable, having no actual direct link to not doing that procedure. Yet the cardiologist remained influenced by it in his or her daily decisions for over-treatment. Other cardiologists in the study had grandiose notions that since heart disease deaths have decreased over recent decades it must be because of the stent procedures they do (and ignore factors such as heart bypass surgery advances, new drug therapies and lifestyle improvements).

When a patient undergoes a heart angiogram to visualize the heart-feeding arteries, if a modest blockage is identified a stent will usually be inserted after scraping open the blockage. This is done despite knowing it may not be helpful to do so. What is more concerning, this iffy procedure will be done *without* a risk-benefit discussion between doctor, patient and family *before* proceeding to the stent treatment. Not all blockages require balloon procedures to open them. Both diagnosis and treatment are usually done consecutively despite lack of benefit for people with stable heart disease (as opposed to those having a heart attack). During this focus group study, cardiologists made comments such as, "He's already gotten to the cath (catheterization) lab" and "There is no chance of escaping." Another key factor influencing cardiologists' decisions to perform angioplasty is fear of malpractice for inaction. When patients convey to doctors their expectations for getting the procedure, it can sway a doctor to recommend angioplasty. These patients with milder heart disease may never find out that risky procedure offered no advantage over taking medications and improving lifestyle.

Technology advances also contribute to over-action by cardiologists, according to the study. As stents and equipment have improved, the complication rate has gone down. This gives cardiologists "license" to stent many blockages unnecessarily since there is less chance for a complication "coming back to bite" them, as one cardiologist phrased it in this study.

Clearly, true and accurate informed consent is hard to attain when doctors who will do the procedure have emotional, egotistical, financial or other misguided motivations for performing that risky procedure.

Here are some lessons to be learned and key points to bear in mind:

1. Second Opinion Rules: Precisely because any given doctor can recommend a procedure for reasons other than best interest of the patient, a second and perhaps third opinion is mandatory before undergoing a risky procedure or operation. Your primary care provider is unlikely to "overrule" a cardiologist's or surgeon's judgment to perform a procedure so the opinion of another objective specialist is necessary in addition to your family doctor's opinion. Do *not* get a second-opinion recommendation from the first cardiologist since that second specialist may well have work by the same aggressive approach. Ask your primary care doctor to recommend a specialist for another opinion, though insurance network limitations can be an obstacle. Needless to say, emergency situations with life at stake will usually not allow for second opinions.
2. Angioplasty with stent placement should *not* be routinely done at the same time as the angiogram that first finds some modest blockages in *stable* heart disease situations. This delay from diagnosis to performing a treatment procedure would allow time for patients to research the risks versus benefits, discuss with doctors the findings and their true implications, and see how their heart is feeling with medical treatment and lifestyle improvement. The down side, of course, is a possible need to schedule a second procedure — a small price to pay since many people likely would opt *against* ever undergoing that questionable angioplasty procedure. As a rule with stable heart disease, unless during a life-threatening crisis, avoid getting invasive treatments at the same time as the test that finds an "abnormality." Take time to research whether a treatment is necessary. Take a watch and wait approach, or perhaps

allow time for safer and simpler treatment alternatives such as lifestyle changes to work.

3. One key missing link in the chain of informed consent is adequate mention of treatment *alternatives* that are given less attention and formal study. Patients usually are offered misleading either-or options: take medications or get no treatment; undergo a procedure or "ignore" the problem; agree to a procedure or you must take several pills. These either-or scenarios are, in a sense, false choices. Either take the drug or risk a stroke. Undergo a stent procedure or suffer a heart attack. Not true! Diet, exercise, stress reduction and other lifestyle modifications can be options that are rarely studied head-to-head against procedures or medical therapies. When those lifestyle changes *have* been carefully studied, as with the diabetes drug, metformin, versus lifestyle changes for heart attack risk, lifestyle improvements convincingly won that contest. In addition, several studies have found the "DASH" diet to lower blood pressure more effectively than medication. Furthermore, the Mediterranean diet can reduce stroke and heart attack risk by 30 percent in healthy folks compared to only a 25 percent relative risk reduction from cholesterol-lowering drugs. The only side effects from the diet treatment are a full stomach and sleepy, content feeling after eating.

First, Clarify Your Personal Goals

Consider the case of a 70 year-old man who suffers from many serious ailments including bleeding and clotting tendencies and diabetes. He has suffered from crippling back problems that have now led to loss of function in one leg, rendering him hunched and wheelchair-bound. A surgeon has scheduled him for surgery to fuse some vertebrae in his back. There remains concern about his ill-defined blood disorders. He may never walk again due to leg nerve damage. His pain is controlled with pain medication. The first question this man must ask is, "What are my key life goals?" His chances to walk again are reduced. Is it for pain relief? If so, can the surgeon give assurance the pain will significantly improve from the surgery? This is unlikely since back surgery frequently does not resolve pain. If this man can have quality of life while dependent upon a wheelchair, and get effective pain relief from medication, then why undergo such risky surgery? Life and death are at stake. Did the surgeon estimate a risk for death from the surgery? Does the surgeon really know since this man has several undefined ailments? Is it worth dying on the table for small potential gains? On the other hand, if the surgery would enable the man to walk again and ambulation is essential to his quality of life, then the surgery might be worth the risk.

Additional personality factors to consider are how motivated someone is to take daily pills or perhaps to exercise and change dietary habits instead of taking medication.

Second Opinion: Can You Trust One Doctor's Conclusions?

You meet a specialist for the first time and he or she tells you the best medical evidence argues you should have that operation or risky procedure. Is the specialist correct? Are there hidden personal reasons why that doctor recommends a procedure? Is the "best evidence" upon which the specialist or primary care doctor bases an opinion truly reliable and accurate? Has the doctor even carefully analyzed the studies? Do they simply make recommendations based upon sometimes biased published guidelines created by so-called experts who commonly have conflicts of interest to promote certain treatments? Dr John Ioannidis, Professor of Health Research and Policy, and Director of the Stanford Prevention Research Center at Stanford University School of Medicine, has argued in his published essay titled, *Why Most Published Research Findings are False*, that a majority of currently published studies are either biased or inaccurate. Dr. Ioannidis also writes, "Currently, many published research findings are false or exaggerated, and an estimated 85% of research resources are wasted."

It is frightening that these same biased studies are what doctors must rely upon to form medical opinions and recommendations for their patients. Here we have a case of too many cooks in the kitchen may be a *good* thing. Second or third opinions with differing perspectives can help slice through some of the bias and exaggeration. Personal biases such as financial gain, emotion-based decisions, accepted overly-aggressive practice patterns in a particular hospital or region, and malpractice fears might be diluted when more than one opinion is considered. In fact, a 2015 study published in the *American Journal of Medicine* offered second opinions for nearly 2700 survey participants. The second opinions resulted in change of diagnosis about 15 percent of the time and change in treatment in nearly 40 percent of cases! Considering a population-based study has estimated that at least one in 20 United States adults are misdiagnosed, and half of these miscues can be harmful, getting more than one cook in the kitchen involved in diagnosing your ailment is surely a wise practice. Clearly, people must be wary of the "medical magic wand effect." This magical and wishful thinking leads patients to believe that any treatment or procedure will help their illness: Any treatment must be better than no treatment, many folks believe. Nothing can be further from the truth. Treatments can be and often are worse than the disease (see chapter).

Folks may be asking themselves right about now:

"How do I know what to ask a doctor before undergoing tests or treatments?"

"Who am I to question a medical expert?"

"How can I even think straight to ask probing questions? The doctor may have just told me I need surgery for cancer or might have suffered a stroke or heart attack, for instance."

These are all valid concerns, which is why I have put together the following **Informed Consent Question Kits (IC-Q- Kits)** to properly prepare folks on how to ask pertinent questions when the fogged mind enters shut-down mode. To take it one step further, I have added IC-Q-Kits for the following key situations:

- When your doctor prescribes new medications: drugs pose grande-sized risks.
- Referral to the emergency room and the many hidden dangers lurking behind those metal doors.
- Referral to see a specialist, or to get a consult from one while you are laid up on a hard emergency room stretcher. A reminder: Specialist consults usually give rise to more tests and procedures, and thus more risks. When serious illness is in question, of course, specialists can become your best ally.

- If hospital admission may be necessary, either as an urgency or electively.

These are situations in which informed consent is virtually nonexistent. A doctor says take this drug and patients fill the prescription. Patients are usually informed with a two-sentence admonition given in the five seconds before the doctor darts out the door. "Go to the emergency room if you are sick." No actual evaluation first. No real discussion of risks, benefits and alternatives. How do you know if the doctor simply fears medical liability or does not want his schedule interrupted by your ailment? That is hardly medical justification to put you through a stressful and risky emergency room visit. Following are lists of key questions to ask your doctor before agreeing to procedures, risky tests, medications, hospitalization, specialist consultation or an emergency room visit.

Many people are intimidated by doctors and are reluctant to question their decisions. Others believe their doctor or other provider will get angry with them if they show skepticism. It is almost reflexive for the mind to go blank after receiving scary news. The **solution:** These IC-Q-Kits will become available as wallet-sized cards to hand to your doctor. These questions serve as insulation from your doctor's quick-fix advice. If the doctor will not take the time to answer these on-point and relevant questions, perhaps the doctor should not be ordering those tests, treatments or medications. Perhaps the doctor does not actually have a deep enough understanding of the health issues and is making rote, poorly thought-out medical decisions on your behalf for all the wrong reasons.

It is too easy for a provider to write a prescription for medication or a diagnostic test to quickly end a visit. A reflexive referral to the emergency room is no sweat for the provider or doctor but a major hardship for patients. The emergency room referral eliminates decision pressure, liability concerns, time constraints, and schedule disruption for the doctor. You, along with your "Patient Power," can make that process a bit harder for the doctor. Cramp the doctor's style a little bit. Your life may be at stake! Hand the doctor a list of questions to answer to slow down that reflexive decision-making. Force the doctor to think about the actual evidence for or against that recommendation, how it affects your individual needs and situation, and what alternatives exist such as watchful waiting. Probing questions can also help to remind the doctor about what is important to you. Remember, too, that a second opinion is always wise before undergoing major tests, treatments, procedures or surgery.

IC-Q-Kit (Informed Consent Question Kit) for Procedures or Surgery

Dear Doctor,

1. Is this surgery or procedure necessary now or can we try safer, non-invasive treatments first? How long can we wait for improvement with safer treatments?
2. What are the most *serious* risks like death or heart attack and how likely are they to occur? Name two or three most *common* risks?
3. Would you object to me getting a second opinion?
4. How many of these procedures have you personally performed? Are there any doctors available who have done pioneering work and specialize in doing mostly the procedure or surgery that I will need?
5. Are less risky procedures available to treat my problem? For instance, less invasive laser or endoscopic approaches rather than major open surgery for a slipped disk?
6. If you still recommend I proceed with the surgery, can you guarantee a high likelihood of success curing my disease, fixing my disability or eliminating my pain? What percent success, failure or serious complications? Any reliable medical studies to support this guarantee?
7. Will the procedure require general anesthesia? Would local or spinal anesthesia be possible and safer? Or perhaps intravenous sedating medication? Do you know the anesthesiologist and is he or she highly skilled for this type of procedure?
8. Do both the surgeon and anesthesiologist accept my insurance plan?

IC-Q-Kit for Medication Prescriptions

Dear Doctor,

1. What specific major studies or reviews of several clinical trials (meta-analyses) support using this medication for my illness and situation? Have medical journals published any expert critiques having concerns about the quality of the study? Are there any unflattering reports on the drug's safety or effectiveness?
2. Is this drug a newly approved medication or one that has been around for many years? It is usually safer to take time-tested medications proven safe and effective over decades of use.
3. "Mathematical significance does *not* equal clinical significance" so how much will I personally benefit? Are the major studies relevant to my sex, age group, or specific chronic illnesses? Population-based studies and results do *not* necessarily apply to me personally.
4. How might this drug affect my quality of life – both negatively or positively?
5. Please explain benefits and risks for me taking this drug in terms of simple numbers. For example, for every 100 people who take this medication everyday to prevent stroke, how many will still have a stroke *while taking* the pill and how many will not? Out of 100 people, how many will NOT have a stroke even *without ever taking* that drug? As an example, blood thinners can help prevent stroke for people who have an irregular heart rhythm called atrial fibrillation. Taking daily blood thinners for years, about 98 percent of people will *not* suffer a stroke. Pretty impressive. However, 96 percent of people *not taking* the drug will also *not* suffer a stroke. Side effects, however, can be serious for people taking the blood thinner thus negating any benefits.
6. What are the more serious side effects from taking this drug? Most common side effects? Any *black box warnings* that might place me at risk for very serious side effects?
7. Have any respected studies been done that show similar benefits from better diet or exercise and other lifestyle changes? If so, are the benefits comparable to taking medication? Shouldn't we first emphasize this nondrug approach? For instance, many studies on diets such as DASH and Mediterranean have shown success in reducing or preventing serious disease like high blood pressure,

diabetes and high cholesterol comparable to or exceeding benefits of drug treatment.

8. Any conflict of interest to report? Do you consult for the drug company that manufactures this medication? Do you receive samples and information, or food or other gifts, from company drug reps?

IC-Q-Kit for Tests Ordered by Your Doctor

Dear Doctor,

1. Is this test really necessary or can it wait a few days to weeks? Maybe my problem will resolve on its own? Are there safer testing options that we can start with if a test must be done now?
2. What key information will the test show? Will that information *change* my treatment plan? For instance, if my back has been hurting for four weeks but I wisely will not rush to have surgical procedures done, why undergo an MRI now? I plan to give it the recommended three months to improve whether or not I have a slipped disk. This assumes there are no signs of cancer like weight loss or disabling pain.
3. What are the risks of undergoing this test? Any radiation? If so, how much — equal to how many chest x-rays? Any cancer risk? Any contrast dye that can cause allergic reactions or kidney damage?
4. What are the risks of watchful waiting without testing for now? Can we give my ailment a few days to improve with simple remedies?
5. Is defensive medicine and liability concern at play in your decision to order this test? If so, and the test is not truly needed, I will gladly sign a "refused testing" note for the chart. I want only tests that are crucial for making a diagnosis of serious illness, if there is a strong likelihood of me having that disease.
6. How likely is it this test will find unexpected "spots" that can be normal body variations that may lead to even riskier testing? For example, most mammogram abnormalities are *not* cancerous,

but these irregularities lead to invasive biopsies and many sleepless nights. As many as 20 percent of breast cancer pathology reports, in fact, are changed when a second opinion is sought by an expert pathologist.

7. Any conflict of interest to report? Do you earn or generate extra income for yourself or your practice by ordering additional tests?

IC-Q-Kit for Emergency Room Referral

Dear Doctor,

1. Is my condition imminently life-threatening so I must go to an emergency room now? Which dangerous ailment are you most worried about and how likely am I to have it (very likely, medium, small chance)?
2. What specifically will doctors do at the emergency room that cannot be done as an outpatient over the next day or two while I get simple treatments and wait for improvement?
3. Are there any other options for me if my condition is not immediately life-threatening? Can you or a specialist squeeze me in for a visit today? Urgent care evaluation? Can you order some treatments and we can give it one or two days to improve? If worse, I will call 911. Is "hospital at home" treatment an option in which you order intravenous treatment for me in my home or assisted living?
4. If not life-threatening, can you see me urgently to help me avoid the hospital visit?
5. If the treating doctor is unfamiliar with you personally, ask how risky it would be to start simple treatment now and wait a day until I can speak to or see my usual primary care provider?
6. If I must go to the ER, will the referring doctor speak to the emergency room doctor about my situation? What diagnosis or two are you most worried about that I may have?
7. Which type of emergency department should I rush to? Teaching hospital? Community hospital? Is there a special chest pain or stroke unit nearby? Geriatric specialty emergency room? Trauma

center? Would a freestanding emergency room or urgent care be able to handle my problem?

IC-Q-Kit for Hospital Admission Recommendation

Dear Doctor,

1. Must I go to the hospital for this illness? What will they do in-hospital that cannot be arranged for me on the outside? Is my ailment imminently life threatening?
2. For frail seniors: Please remember that I am at high risk for many complications and loss of function if I go to the hospital. Can "hospital at home" be arranged for less complicated ailments so I can get needed treatment in my house, care home or assisted living facility? This could reduce my risk for hospital-acquired infections, adverse drug events, inadequate nutrition, bedsores and function loss.
3. Perhaps I can get some intravenous treatments and needed testing in the emergency room and then get home health care or infusion services at home rather than staying in the hospital?
4. Perhaps I can get basic treatment now and I will see my primary care doctor within a day or two for follow up care.
5. Is defensive medicine or liability fear at play in the decision to hospitalize me? If so, I will gladly sign a waiver indicating I refused your advice to be hospitalized.
6. If I must be hospitalized, can you admit me directly onto a floor ward? How long can I expect to be in the hospital? Can someone drive me or must I call 911?
7. If I must go to the hospital via the emergency room, will you notify the ER to let them know I am arriving? Which doctor do you suggest I see at the emergency department? Can you forward a few relevant records and my presumptive diagnosis to ER staff?

IC-Q-Kit for Referral to a Specialist

Dear Doctor,

1. Do I really need to see a specialist? Specialist referrals are most important for undergoing necessary procedures that primary care doctors do not perform. For instance, colonoscopy to investigate rectal bleeding. A specialist may also be necessary to try to diagnose or treat complex illness after basic evaluations are completed by your family doctor or ER doctor.
2. Can the specialist do anything for me that does not involve risky tests, treatments or drugs? If I prefer holding off on these risky treatments, is there anything more we can try that is safe and effective?
3. If I must see a specialist, can you refer me to one with specific expertise for my specific problem? We are now in the era of sub-sub-specialist care.
4. I prefer seeing a specialist affiliated with a specific hospital system with a fine reputation. Can you get me into that system?
5. Will my insurance cover that specialist referral in-network?
6. How long can my problem wait until I get an appointment with that specialist? Should you call and speak to the specialist to arrange for prompt evaluation or to share your concerns? Otherwise, will you forward my relevant records to the specialist?

A Few Eye-Popping Facts and Statistics:

- Three-quarters of general practitioners admitted having problems understanding statistics commonly found in medical journals, according to one study. If the doctor lacks informed understanding, how can he or she offer to patients true informed consent?
- Doctors may not appreciate this tenet relevant to medical studies: "Effectiveness at the group level may mean uncertainty at the individual level."
- True informed consent involves an ongoing process by which doctor and patient exchange information, questions and opinions about benefits and risks for any significant care recommendation.
- Medical professionals should offer support and distill complex

medical information and uncertainty into crystal clear and unbiased options for best patient care. Several different options with pros and cons should be discussed. The patient can now choose an approach most in keeping with his or her personal needs and wishes. This, and only this, is person-centered care.

- Fleeting doctor-patient encounters in all settings are a setup for lack of true informed consent. A ten-minute visit simply cannot include proper informed consent discussion about tests, treatments, medications or anything, really.
- How doctors **frame** an issue can be critical in how a patient chooses from several options. For instance, patients are more likely to undergo a risky angioplasty procedure, for instance, if the doctor says, "The procedure has a 97 percent chance for success" as opposed to "Of 100 people who undergo the angioplasty, one will die and two will suffer serious complications from the procedure such as hemorrhage, stroke or heart attack."
- Overly detailed information does not necessarily translate into greater understanding by patients. After a while, complex information sounds like the doctor is speaking Swahili. None of it will register.
- Based upon recent informed consent court decisions, doctors are required to disclose *all risks* that might affect someone's decision for or against a treatment or procedure. Key elements of informed consent include a patient who is *competent* to make decisions and give *voluntary* consent; a diagnosis that requires the treatment plan in question; nature and description of procedure or treatment being offered; expected results; reasonable alternative treatment options, including risks or benefits of not doing any treatment; potential risks and complications versus expected benefits of the treatment or procedure; explanation of any uncertainties about the treatment; an assessment whether the patient understands the plan presented. Conflicts of interest and financial gain that might affect a doctor's decision to proceed with a procedure or treatment should also be disclosed to patients. There is also legal precedent obligating physicians to disclose their expertise or lack thereof with

a specific procedure since that could significantly affect outcome and a decision to move forward with the procedure. An exception to full informed consent does exist if disclosing too much information poses a threat to a patient's emotional health.

DANGER 9. PLANNING YOUR LAST WISHES: DON'T WORRY, DIE HAPPY

I'm not afraid of death; I just don't want to be there when it happens.

Woody Allen

The fear of death follows from the fear of life. A man who lives fully is prepared to die at any time.

Mark Twain

While I thought that I was learning how to live, I have been learning how to die.

Leonardo da Vinci

I am prepared to meet my Maker. Whether my Maker is prepared for the great ordeal of meeting me is another matter.

Winston Churchill

No pioneering procedure or designer drug will undo our telomeric destiny.

*Sometimes, death is **not** optional.*

Joel Cohen

Would you create your plan for a fire drill while the house is burning down? Is it wise to formulate your strategy for health emergencies while you already feel that elephant sitting on your chest? Similarly, preparing to "die happy" – in a way you choose and that fits your personal wishes – should not be formulated or finalized *after* crisis strikes or bad news of serious illness arrives. Folks should certainly not devise a "Die-Happy Plan" when death looms near. The haze and fog of illness are opaque, with clear vision obscured by confusion, pain, mind-altering medications and searing emotion. Furthermore, each individual must face the simple truth that nobody else can plan or bring to fruition for you a "happy death", not even close friends or loved ones. Death is too personal and intimate. Implementing a plan for dying happy cannot be outsourced.

Each individual has unique spiritual needs and religious beliefs. Many people, however, look the other way, like an unprepared child in reading class, and hope the Grim Reaper will not call upon them. Fear of death might be alleviated by facing it head on and with a smile. As they say, the most common cause of death is... life. Death is the final stage of living and should be done right. One can curl up in a corner, cowering and trembling with fear and anticipating its arrival. Or one may choose to ponder and plan a "happy death" that is in keeping with one's spiritual, religious and philosophical wishes and values.

A person cannot pick and choose when and how he or she dies. Some die softly during slumber; others must stare down dreaded discomfort and pain. But preparation can help to enhance the inevitable death experience. Perhaps more important, less suffering during one's dying process translates into reduced trauma, guilt and pain for loved ones as well. If someone fears death less, or embraces it, loved ones may be spared much angst. Family and friends might also learn by example what courage looks like.

First, get the finances squared away. Craft a Last Will & Testament and Living Will and assign at least two healthcare surrogates (decision makers) – primary and backup – in case you lose your ability to choose your own choices. These accounting and legal details, however, are insufficient to achieve a happy death. One must strive to heal key relationships; find sense of purpose; pursue dreams and goals; seek and offer forgiveness where appropriate; and leave a legacy of wishes, values and accomplishments – all key components of fully living as well as ingredients for happy dying. This long and layered process and journey must begin now... today. How many tomorrows remain?

Which death scenario would you prefer?

Your heart stops in a sterile white room filled with dispassionate strangers. Your nude, still body is on display like a manikin at a department store as doctors and nurses jab it with needles and insert tubes into every orifice. Squealing alarms and piercing beeps fill the room above the chanted orders and chatter. Some of those strangers dressed in scrubs begin pumping on your chest and cracking and snapping your ribs. A few 300-Joule electrical zaps to your chest jolt your body a few inches off the hard stretcher, despite little hope for igniting an old and stalled heart. With CPR, death comes like a jackhammer ripping into worn concrete. In the end, chances for an old, ill person to survive chest compressions and its accompaniments are slim to none. Those whose hearts are reignited often spend weeks in intensive care, hooked up to machines until death.

Or do you prefer calming violin music soothing your soul? Flowery scents wafting through the room – perhaps lavender or peppermint? Your favorite artwork or photos surround you in a familiar environment of your own choosing. A morphine haze numbs your pain, allowing peaceful slumber. Reassuring words from family and friends remind you how much you are loved. Tender hand-holding from those who matter most allow for final goodbyes. Simple touching has never felt so good. You are grinning from the Grim Reaper's feathery tickle.

The choice is yours. You *can* decide.

Avoidable Suffering: Letting Loved Ones Go

Mr. H breathed like a puffer fish as his lips pursed and cheeks bellowed out to compensate for damaged lungs, ravaged from a lifetime of smoking. As a war veteran, his eyes lit up any time he told his doctor about past war stories. Back then, he was strong and in control, but not now. His atrophied muscles and scarred lungs forced daily dependency. He well understood his poor prognosis and in discussing end-of-life care, he and his children agreed he wanted to have a better death than the bad experience his wife had recently suffered in her final days. Mr. H's wife died hard in the hospital so he made his wishes clear he did not want to go to an emergency room or hospital under any circumstances.

With home visits to Mr. H's well-kept house every couple of months, his doctor managed to alleviate his shortness of breath and anxiety. After a year of juggling medications and reassurance, Mr. H suddenly took a turn for the worse. He appeared to be struggling more to breathe and was confused during a house call visit. His oxygen level cratered more than usual on the next visit. Perhaps his emphysema was finally winning the battle. He was weaker, more confused and gasping with each breath. His pufferfish complexion changed from red to ghost-white.

The family agreed to use hospice services despite reluctance based upon the wife's negative experience. Mr. H continued his decline but his children voiced concern that perhaps the doctor should be doing more to evaluate why he had deteriorated. To his doctor, it seemed clear his lungs were ravaged by emphysema scarring – a terminal disease. His children pressured the doctor to order blood tests. A surprising result: a very low red blood cell count (anemia) which might have contributed to his deterioration. Most likely though, the anemia resulted *from* his unavoidable decline. The house call doctor convinced hospice nurses to arrange for a two-pint blood transfusion to assuage family concerns and to hopefully alleviate Mr. H's air hunger. He only slid deeper into a breathing abyss. A few days later, while at home with his children, his panicked daughter called 911 when Mr. H appeared to be on death's door.

His worst fears were realized. Off Mr. H went by ambulance to the hospital despite his many conversations with his doctor and insistence he be spared that suffering. His doctor had long conversations with family members about his imminently terminal condition and they seemed to recognize this fact. When the doctor mentioned morphine for comfort care as the only option remaining, the sick man's daughter blurted out, "I know he's just another GOMER to you! That's why you won't do anything for him!"

GOMER is a derogatory term used more commonly in the past to describe mostly sick, older patients with little hope for recovery with whom doctors wanted little interaction. This was a shocking comment for Mr. H's doctor who provided nothing but quality and compassionate care to him.

The anecdote above is a summary of Dr. David Muller's essay published in *Health Affairs* journal based upon his own experiences. Dr. Muller made the following insightful statement in his essay:

For any given patient, a doctor might have to take into account different opinions, different personalities, and a lifetime of complicated family dynamics. This requires skills that aren't taught in medical school... Doctors can play a crucial role in orchestrating a "good" death, but they can also—despite the best of intentions—be a party to a miserable one.

How did it all end for Mr. H? Dr. Muller describes the details in his essay:

Mr. H languished in the hospital for more than a month after that bedside family meeting... He was delirious every minute of every day, hungry for air, bedbound, incontinent, and often restrained. He finally died when there was nothing left of him.

The moral is simple: All of the world's hi-tech medical care cannot make death optional. Doctors and their families must strive to honor a person's wishes for a happy death — whichever way each individual envisions it to be. When the body comes undone, quality of life, dignity and personal choice to die one's own way, on one's own terms, and in one's chosen setting is all a person has left. A person's spirit, memory and legacy are all that will remain.

The following anecdote illustrates the importance of **death acceptance** and allowing time to say goodbye to seriously ill loved ones:

This "cat" may have had only three lives. He was 67-year-old Terence Foley who was diagnosed seven years earlier with kidney cancer. As his wife describes in her eloquent essay published in Bloomberg Business Week Magazine in 2010, she describes Terence as a fighter who played fifteen musical instruments and recently had earned a doctorate. After two previous brushes with death, now the cancer had spread to his lungs. Over the years Terence and his wife struggled through fierce battles, trying every new drug that showed any benefit against cancers including Interleukin and Avastin. Perhaps they would be the cure? Perhaps they would only buy a few treasured weeks or months? But were the treatments worth it?

"Some drugs Terence took probably did him no good. At least one (drug)

helped fewer than 10 percent of patients," Mrs. Foley writes in her essay. This implies that 90 percent of patients treated with this drug are subjected to serious side effects, suffering and cost – all for naught.

After her husband's drawn-out death, during which he was subjected to many potent treatments and side effects, Mrs. Foley visited the oncologist. She writes: *"Did we help Terence or harm him? There's a possibility, (the oncologist) said, that the treatment actually made the cancer worse, causing it to rage out of control at the end. Or, as another doctor suggested in passing at the time, the strokes (he suffered from) were a side effect of the Sutent (a new drug) and not the cancer."*

Hope and optimism are crucial ingredients to healing. But each person and family, during their serious illness journey, must come to terms with that unspoken possibility that the end might finally be near. Letting go is hard for family, but easier for those who are infirm and suffer. Signs the end is near can be striking: a sudden and rapid deterioration after prolonged illness; a major setback or event like a stroke; lost function such as becoming fully bedridden; cyclical rapid breathing followed by a long pause; reduced alertness and inability to communicate; new confusion; cold hands; grayish or sallow skin color; and persistent rattling in the chest with each breath.

Affirming that death is near is as important as hope and optimism. Preparations must be made. Friends and relatives must be notified to allow them time to travel. The key process of saying goodbye can only be possible with acceptance of death. Mrs. Foley offers critical insight into her own experience:

"Looking back, memories of my zeal to treat are tinged with sadness. Should I have given up earlier? Would earlier hospice care been kinder? I hadn't believed Terence was going to die so I had never confronted any of those dilemmas. And I never let us have the chance to say goodbye."

Mary's Last Request Ignored

Mary stared at the ceiling in the intensive care unit, startled by beeping monitors and alarms. Only that plastic tube stuffed down her throat stopped her from screaming. Mary's spunk and free spirit had not waned even after eighty years. She ignored doctors who for forty years warned her to give up her two vices – smoking and drinking. Mary outlived them all. That day, she arrived at the emergency room gasping for air. Her lips were blue, skin ashen, flabby muscles fatigued and heart weary. Emphysema and heart failure had caught up with Mary. She grimaced and waved the doctor away, but was too winded to speak. The emergency room doctor had seen many such 'combative' patients struggling to breathe. Mary's arms flailed, trying to stop the inevitable. The doctor brushed off her gestures and injected an intravenous sedative. A soporific haze quieted Mary's protests while the doctor inserted a breathing tube into her windpipe. The nurse connected a ventilator to give Mary the breathing help she desperately did not want.

Mary's lungs filled with air like inflating party balloons. Silently, she told herself she could never forgive the emergency room doctor for saving her life. She had signed a "Do Not Resuscitate" or DNR form because she decided long ago she wished to die gracefully, the way she had lived. She would not be kept alive by noisy machines. She wanted no part of those intensive care units where she would not be permitted to smoke or drink. She had heard about the cracking and crunching of ribs, and poking and prodding with tubes and needles, when CPR is performed. Even with that barbaric ritual, CPR has a very low success rate, she was told. Mary never let anybody tell her what to do during her lifetime. "Sure won't let doctors and nurses pound on my chest when I die," she once said. With a chuckle she added, "The day I die is the one day in my life I'd like to have some peace and quiet."

It is not uncommon for Do Not Resuscitate paperwork and last wishes to be overlooked and misunderstood when someone is rushed by ambulance to an emergency room. In fact, too often family is unprepared and neglects to complete the required documents for each state or country to order healthcare workers to follow last wishes. They mistakenly rely on vague language in a Living Will, but paramedics and emergency professionals neither read nor see Living Wills. What's more, those legal documents are *not* actual medical orders that would guide decisions by doctors during medical crises. The ER doctor must then act quickly and might inadvertently perform extraordinary procedures against the patient's wishes when life or death hangs in the balance. Mary suffered for several weeks with tubes down her throat, no cigarettes or alcohol, and a wilting and harsh decline as death lumbered in to her rescue. She did not realize that a DNR order applies specifically *after* the heart and breathing stop, not while someone is still alive. She should have been more specific with *pre-death* end of life wishes. Mary had always celebrated life, but her final days were no party.

The process of creating a happy death takes years of planning, introspection, and discussion with doctors, spiritual advisors, loved ones and friends.

Layers of a Happy Death: It is EEEEasy, Sort of

Explore: Read about death, religion, philosophy and how they affect your personal wishes. Absorb and ponder experiences with dying pets, sickly grandparents, and other medical illnesses, tragedies and deaths. A few must watch movies: The truth-based movie titled, *Tuesdays with Morrie*; animated masterpiece titled *Up*; *The Bucket List*; *The Notebook*; *My Life*.

Must reading: For a more complete picture of decisions that must be considered in completing a "Die-Happy" Plan, read the following materials that are available online, just a small sampling of available vast and rich resources to learn more:

- POLST Form – Available in 16 states and counting. California, Oregon, Montana, Washington State, Utah, Idaho, Colorado, Iowa, Louisiana, Tennessee, New York, West Virginia, Pennsylvania, Hawaii, Georgia, North Carolina
- Your State or Country's Do Not Resuscitate form, or equivalent
- Durable Power of Attorney for Healthcare or Healthcare Proxy forms (substitute decision maker)
- Five Wishes document from agingwithdignity.org
- The many books on death and dying by Elizabeth Kubler Ross, a renowned psychiatrist and researcher on this subject
- *How We Die: Reflections of Life's Final Chapter*, by Dr. Sherwin B. Nuland

Explain: Discuss with family, friends, spiritual advisors and healthcare providers your personal wishes regarding death based upon your readings and experiences. Explain your wishes verbally and in writing. Family members may be forced to make heart-wrenching care decisions that should be based upon *your* clearly expressed wishes, not their wish to keep you alive another day or week. What would you like your death experience to be like?

- Death at home versus in a hospital, hospice facility or skilled care facility
- Your Ideal "Dying Room:" Flowers; scents; music; presence of specific friends, loved ones and spiritual advisors; art or photos to be displayed; individuals you do *not* want present
- Before the final event arrives, personal messages you would like to convey to friends or family such as advice, apology, forgiveness, legacy or final promise (verbally, in writing or on video)
- Treasured possessions you would like around you or that you wish to personally bequeath to loved ones
- Treasured activities you would like to do (if possible, as tolerated) in your final weeks of life such as visiting the ocean or forest, speaking to someone not seen for years, watching sunsets, seeing a concert, or any other whimsical but attainable goal
- Simple pleasures you would like more of; anything distasteful to you to be avoided
- Burial, cremation or donation of body to science or organ donation; place of burial or body donation
- Funeral ceremony or other memorial service; happy and upbeat versus sad and mournful
- Poem, essay, quotes, or message you will want read or conveyed at your ceremony
- Specific music or song to be played

Elaborate: Work with a legal consultant to develop an Advance Directive or Living Will based upon local laws and requirements in your state or country. Also designate a durable power of attorney or healthcare proxy (substitute decision maker) and a backup decision maker. These proxies should be well-acquainted with your philosophies and wishes on dying since they will make final decisions about your care if you no longer can.

Be certain they will not extend your *dying process* to "keep you around longer" unless that is specifically your wish.

Expand and implement plan: This part is especially important to implement if you suffer from serious disease or chronic ailments, physical disability, frailty or terminal illness. There are, of course, two types of terminal illness: The first is *active* terminal illness such as untreatable advanced cancer with a life prognosis under a few months; the second is *chronic* terminal illness such as heart failure, emphysema, Parkinson's disease, progressive multiple sclerosis, Lou Gehrig's disease and dementia. These terminal diseases can fester for five to ten years or more and are usually accompanied by episodes of sudden medical crises requiring hospitalization, temporary recovery, and then progressive deterioration.

Now would be a good time to read the Five Wishes document, POLST orders form, Do Not Resuscitate order form and whether your Living Will instructions are specific and clear. Your Living Will should also define quality of life red lines past which you would not want to extend life any more if all meaning and quality has been lost (see below).

Quality of Life Red Lines

It is crucial for people to define what losses in function or quality of life would make continued living a burden to them and their family, based upon their own values and spiritual or philosophical beliefs. At this point, they would want either:

1. Only comfort care without tubes or procedures to prolong life; No medication treatment other than for pain and suffering
2. Comfort care plus antibiotic treatment and other necessary medications
3. Hospitalization or emergency room treatment if needed, without procedures or surgeries
4. Hospitalization or emergency room treatment plus necessary procedures and surgeries

The Quality of Life Red Lines (check any that apply to you, circle care wishes 1, 2, 3, or 4 if red line crossed by succumbing to that condition):

□ **Comatose**, with little or no chance for meaningful recovery based upon two specialist opinions

1. Comfort Care only **2**. Comfort Care Plus medications **3**. Hospital or ER, No procedures **4**. Hospital or ER, Plus necessary procedures or surgery

□ **Non-Communicative** and unable to communicate with loved ones either verbally, with eye contact, emotional responses, hugs, or no apparent facial recognition. This is likely permanent.

1. 2. 3. 4. (see numbered options just above)

□ **Fully Bedridden or Homebound** due to injury (paralysis), brain disease, or medical ailments requiring all-day care to assist with activities of daily living (can still communicate). Includes loss of ability to care for oneself and tend to one's own daily bodily functions. Or cannot visit or see one's children or grandchildren.

1. 2. 3. 4.

□ **Cannot Care for Myself** requiring caregiver assistance most of the time to help me with daily functions such as eating, bathing, dressing, toileting. Incontinence of urine or poop requiring diaper changes. I am extremely independent and would be too humiliated to bear this. If I change my mind in the future after suffering disability, I will inform my loved ones and doctor to change this specific choice of red line.

1. 2. 3. 4.

□ **Severe, Intractable Pain** or discomfort (nausea, air hunger, diarrhea) that has not responded adequately to medication or holistic treatments. Pain or discomfort is present most of the time and prevents me from enjoying activities.

1. 2. 3. 4.

□ **Loss of Higher Mental Functions** or sound mind due to dementia, brain disease or brain injury. If I am unaware, confused or disoriented most of the time and cannot engage in meaningful dialog or productive higher mental function. Cannot read, write, use deductive reasoning or work productively. Cannot think creatively. This is deemed by experts to be irreversible.

1. 2. 3. 4.

□ **My Survival is Dependent Upon Machines**, leading to limited quality of life. For instance, I cannot breathe sufficiently without a ventilator, or require dialysis machines or other devices to sustain life. If I should change my opinion once I get seriously ill, and my quality of life can still be good, then extraordinary technological treatments would be acceptable to me. I would then revise this red line instruction.

□ **Loss of Ability to Eat Food and Joy of Nourishment and Flavor**. Will require artificial nutrition through vein or feeding tube that is likely to be permanent based upon specialist opinion.

1. 2. 3. 4.

□ **Loss of Ability to Read or Write**, or look at photos of loved ones, or browse art books or other cherished books or objects.

1. 2. 3. 4.

□ **Loss of Ability to Watch Television** or listen to music. Sensory isolation from irreversible loss of vision and hearing and perhaps other senses.

1. 2. 3. 4.

□ **Loss of Ability to Connect with Nature** by watching sunsets, or visiting a beach or forest, or helping out in a garden, or consciously smelling the scent of flowers, or seeing animals in nature, or caring for a valued pet such as dog or cat.

1. 2. 3. 4.

□ If I **Must Live in a Skilled Nursing Facility** or Assisted Living Facility, and cannot be mobile and self-sufficient. <u>Caveat</u>: Feelings about this may well change as you get older and more infirm.

1. 2. 3. 4.

□ **Permanently Unable to Recognize Loved Ones**

1. 2. 3. 4.

□ **Any Other Red Line You Feel Would Render Life Meaningless for You Personally**

____

____

1. 2. 3. 4.

Alternatively:

□ **Life is Precious and Should be Prolonged at All Cost** based upon my religious or philosophic beliefs. Do all that is necessary to keep me alive and comfortable.

□ Despite my frail condition, I **Wish to Live a Little Longer** to Attend a valued event or a landmark occasion such as a wedding or birth. Perform more aggressive treatments until after that occasion, then return to comfort care only.

The Procedures: Do or Don't

Following are **Specific Procedures and Life-Prolonging Technology** that I *refuse* if I am sick and frail, diagnosed with terminal illness, or suffer from chronic disease, and at least one of my quality of life red lines has been crossed (I lost valued quality of life for any reason(s) above).

Check any procedures you would **REFUSE** due to loss of your defined quality-of-life red lines:

□ CPR □ ACLS including defibrillation shocks □ Breathing Tube/Ventilator

□ Dialysis □ Heart Pacemaker □ Heart Angioplasty/Catheterization

□ Major Surgery □ Heart Balloon Pump □ Blood Transfusions

□ Lumbar Puncture (spinal tap) □ Hospitalization □ Emergency Room Visit

□ Clot-dissolving drugs for Heart Attack □ Clot-dissolving drugs for Stroke

□ Artificial nutrition, feeding tube in stomach or intestine □ Artificial nutrition through a vein

□ Central (Large) Vein Intravenous Access □ Arterial Puncture

□ Cardiac Care Unit Treatment □ Intensive Care Unit

□ Chemotherapy □ Radiation Therapy

□ Imaging like PET, CT, MRI Scans □ Invasive Tissue Biopsies

□ Any Future Invasive Technologies not yet developed, unless they are curative for my disease, pain or suffering, or can restore to me significant quality of life.

It is important to understand that you *can* elect to try any of the above interventions, dialysis for example, for a specified period of time. If in this case kidney function improves within two weeks then dialysis can be continued until no longer needed. If, on the other hand, kidney function does not get any better, and full dialysis (or other procedure) is still required and will likely be necessary henceforth, then you might want dialysis stopped – if it means losing key quality of life for you. Once again, any decisions you make should be reevaluated every five years and can be adjusted if you have a change of heart or health condition that transforms your point of view.

Die-Happy Process for Folks over Age 45

1. Ponder death. Not with dread but as a final chapter in a complete life chock full of dreams fulfilled, relationships nurtured, and hard work. Balance accomplishments with leisure and down time. Read about death and dying, how death is approached in different cultures and religions, and philosophies of death and dying.
2. Notate what life activities give you meaning and spiritual fulfillment and elevation. Is it practice of religion? Is it walking along a beach at sunset, the salty water caressing your toes? Is it volunteer work? Animal Rescue? Red Cross work? Hiking in a forest and counting animal sightings? Time with family, friends and children that is most cherished? Travel across the globe? Photography? Creative writing? Now act on that list of spiritually uplifting activities you have jotted down. Just do them. Make time now. The journey of life is like walking a path on the shores of the ocean; once a path is forged, no step can ever be retraced for it has changed the moment you stepped forward. Our time here is too precious for regrets.
3. Speak about your impressions of death, fears and concerns. Talk to loved ones, doctors, friends, spiritual advisors. Think about your life experiences with a dying loved one or pet and what affected you most. Start to formulate a list of definite "wants" and "do not wants" that either appeal to your spiritual values or repulse you. For instance, if you watched a grandparent suffer from pain of metastatic cancer perhaps it is pain you fear most at the end of life.

Or you might know somebody who suffered a devastating stroke and feel your life would not have meaning if you could no longer care for yourself or hike or walk on the beach. This might then become your quality of life red line. If crossed, you would place limitations on all or specific extraordinary measures that prolong life. For instance, no dialysis or no breathing machine if your kidneys shut down or breathing ability is compromised.

4. Caveat: With aging and debility, people often adjust their limits and red lines. You can always revise your decisions in the future if you change your mind. Example: That paralyzed leg and arm may seem repulsive now but if paralysis from a stroke strikes you, but you can see your grandchildren who visit you often, perhaps a life in a wheelchair becomes worth living after all. Perhaps not. What if you can still take your motorized scooter to get coffee each morning at the neighborhood café despite paralysis? You must decide based upon your specific needs, goals and circumstances. Refer to the specific red line information earlier in this chapter.

5. Put together a list of goals, dreams and wishes. Try incorporating into your daily life at least one task or goal that is meaningful to you. Also document your thoughts about what you surely would or would not want should *irreversible* medical crisis strike you. These key concepts can be written informally with only loved ones aware they are documented, or can be the start of a formal Living Will. This does not require an attorney to draft, but it would be prudent to check online for any specific regulations your state or country requires.

6. Consider who could serve as your substitute decision-maker if you lost capacity. Usually a child, spouse, sibling or close friend. You will need a backup healthcare proxy or durable power of attorney for healthcare (informally known as substitute decision maker) in case you outlive your first choice.

7. Live each day caring for your body and soul. Treat your precious body and spirit with the respect they deserve by living well, eating well, avoiding body toxins, and exercising regularly.

8. Ponder your ideal "Death Room." Considerations include dying at

home versus in a hospital setting. Any uplifting scents you would want such as lavender or peppermint or roses? Valued photos or paintings with special meaning? Who would you most want to be present? Let them know and write it down. Perhaps a spiritual advisor, siblings, friends, spouse, children? Would hand-holding and touch be desired? Any special requests such as playing a memory DVD from the past or scenes at an ocean? Any religious rituals or prayers? Music playing? Uplifting or favorite album or classical or somber or chant music?

9. Will you leave a legacy? Any valued messages or keepsakes or treasured items to leave for children or grandchildren? Let people know what goes to whom and where it is kept.

Die-Happy Process for Older Folks with Chronic Illness, their Power of Attorney, or Caregivers of Frail Elderly

Folks who are in the declining health years should perform an accelerated version of the above process for healthy adults, if they still can. But many more complicated issues must be clarified and implemented. End of life care is wholly misunderstood. Many people, as well as doctors, believe that all end-of-life care issues are addressed and solved when they sign a Do Not Resuscitate (DNR or DNAR or NFR) form based upon their Living Will or wishes not to get extraordinary treatments when they are in the declining years. Sadly, this is not what DNR status does. This misunderstanding may lead to an unhappy death if an unexpected situation or status confusion undermines a person's last wishes. The confusion does not come as a surprise since doctors spend just a few minutes discussing a DNR order with patients or their family. This is simply not enough time. Moreover, many doctors mistakenly believe that a DNR order addresses care in the final months to years of life. In truth, it only addresses *what not* to do when someone has died naturally (heart and breathing have suddenly stopped). The American Medical Association Code of Medical Ethics emphasizes that a DNR order should not affect other end-of-life treatment decisions; in other words, the tendency to automatically withhold treatments like transfusions and invasive procedures in folks with a DNR order should be avoided unless specified by each individual (see five care levels below).

What exactly does a DNR form do? One thing and only one — *after* you *die* DNR is an activated official doctor's order to emergency workers to leave you alone. Your heart and/or breathing must have stopped already which means you have died. For old and frail folks, CPR at this point has a slim chance for success anyway. I call DNR "Do Not Reincarnate," meaning once a person has died, do not try to bring them back to life using brutal chest compressions, tubes and machines. The deceased person is not Frankenstein zapped with a bolt of lightning. CPR will rarely help or work under these circumstances, contrary to the 75 percent success rate depicted in movies and television dramas. Completing a DNR form is completely reasonable and appropriate for those in the declining months to years. One recent survey of doctors found that 88 percent of those asked said they would *not* want CPR done on themselves since they are well aware of its brutality and futility in sick, old folks. That says quite a lot. However, the DNR form says nothing about care you wish to have at the end of life, before your heart stops. Choices for end of life care with a signed DNR in place can be wide-ranging and disparate:

Level One

DNR plus comfort care only (perhaps hospice) and no further treatments. Nutrition only if person wishes to and is able to eat or drink. No procedures. No Hospitalization. No dialysis or breathing tube. No operations. Pain, air hunger, nausea, restlessness, spiritual distress, depression and anxiety are the primary goals for treatment.

Level Two

DNR plus comfort care plus simple treatments such as antibiotics for infection, nitroglycerin for chest pain and similar basic medication therapy. No hospitalization, procedures, surgery, artificial nutrition or other extraordinary treatments.

Level Three

DNR plus hospitalization, if needed, to treat such ailments as serious pneumonia, dehydration, abdominal pain, heart attack or any other acute illness not treatable at home, assisted living or skilled nursing. Prefer *not* to have surgery or extraordinary procedures such as dialysis or breathing tube or pacemaker, for instance. Intravenous fluids, feeding and drugs are acceptable (or not, if so specified). Specific procedures that are acceptable or not desired are best spelled out on the DNR form or an addendum page signed by your doctor and stapled to the official state DNR form.

Level Four

DNR plus hospitalization plus all necessary procedures or surgeries required for acute illness that is treatable and likely *reversible*. For instance, pacemaker insertion if the heartbeat peters out. Another example would be accepting a breathing tube and ventilator assistance to treat a serious pneumonia causing breathing failure. The assumption is the new illness will improve with temporary medical support and intravenous antibiotics. Note any treatments you do not want done, for instance dialysis for kidney failure, and specify clearly why you refuse that specific treatment.

Level Five

DNR plus hospitalization plus perform any procedures or surgery that the doctors and your substitute decision maker feel can help prolong life. In other words, "Do everything."

It is unfortunate that most DNR forms have little extra room on them to clarify which level of care you desire *during final months of life* besides not performing CPR once the heart has already stalled. I suggest writing short phrases onto the form in an open space. For longer and more specific information consider typing it onto an "Addendum to DNR" and specifying what your wishes are while still alive (No breathing tube, No hospitalization, No emergency room, no surgery, no feeding tube, etc). Have your doctor sign the addendum below your own signature. **Note:** There is no known legal acceptance for this process I now describe, but it should be honored if the addendum is stapled to the back of the main form and properly signed. The front of the form should clearly note: "read back page too."

Life Review

During the declining years, consider the process of a life review or reminiscence of key events in your life. Write about your successes, failures, dreams fulfilled or those you would like to attain, most meaningful accomplishments and activities, valued relationships you have or wish to mend, and legacy you wish to leave after you are gone.

"Life can only be understood backwards, but it must be lived forwards," wrote philosopher Søren Kierkegaard.

Additional Key Tips and Reminders

- **Living Will:** This document only kicks into action if you are no longer able to or competent to make decisions. Emergency workers, however, will not sit and read your will during an emergency. Your Living Will must be translated into an official DNR or POLST (Physicians Order for Life Sustaining Treatment) medical order that should be honored by medics and doctors. When you write up your wishes in a Living Will, you might want to include that you are of sound mind, clear thought and free of mental illness that could taint your decisions. Add explanations and specific examples of why you choose to get or refuse certain types of care so people know these values are sacred. For instance: "I want everything done to extend my life due to my religious belief that any life is sacred." Alternatively, "I watched my mother suffer through a slow, painful death with loss of her dignity so I would never want to extend life if I am bedridden and mostly dependent on caregivers." Or "I do not want to burden my family the way I endured mental anguish caring for my declining mom." This Living Will document is one that you as individual write up, not necessarily an attorney. Getting it notarized and checking online for any local legal requirements is prudent. In addition, avoid vague statements like "Do not use extraordinary treatment if I am in a coma" as your final summation of wishes unless you want every treatment done in the final months of life. Most people are *not* in a coma until the last few hours to days of life. With new technology and treatments, the period of chronic illness and declining health has been extended significantly – sometimes for a decade or more. NOTE: Do not neglect to specify how much decision-making flexibility your substitute decision-maker should have (use appropriate legal documents also): Follow my living will to the letter, or make care decision adjustments based upon the situation and doctor guidance, or freely make any and all of my care decisions as my disease progresses.

- **DNR form (or DNAR, NFR):** This official order kicks into effect only *after* your heart stops and you have died naturally. It tells healthcare professionals nothing about how extensive or basic you wish your care to be in your declining years (see five levels above). I suggest that you add as much detail as possible to this document regarding major treatments refused or accepted *while still alive* such as 911 activation, feeding tube, breathing tube, dialysis, etc. Caveat: If emergency workers and caregivers do not have immediate access to this paperwork during a crisis, your wishes might be ignored. Make copies of this documentation available to your doctors, substitute decision makers, attorney, caregivers, local paramedics, and hospitals. Keep the original on your refrigerator at home or in your chart if in assisted living or skilled nursing care. Consider using an alert bracelet indicating your DNR status, a requirement in the state of New York. A wallet-sized "Notice in case of accident or other emergency" card placed in your purse or wallet can be helpful at times. Do not forget to search online for specific state or country requirements to satisfy local laws regarding DNR procedures. For instance, some states require an original form only, others allow copies to be legally acceptable. Caveat: If your attorney completed all DNR paperwork in Boston and you have since moved to Florida, your paperwork will need to be redone to conform to local requirements. Note that university and teaching hospitals have an intrinsic culture to treat more aggressively and do more. Studies have found DNR status to be used less commonly at larger academic medical centers.
- **POLST (Physician Orders for Life-sustaining Treatment):** Like DNR, POLST is an official doctor's order to honor wishes to accept or refuse basic treatments such as CPR, aggressive versus

comfort care, and artificial nutritional support. The drawbacks are that it is currently only fully available in 16 states and does not go into detail regarding the many specific advanced treatments that may or may not be acceptable to folks. This document is simple, covers the basics and can be used in the last year or two of life as a simple order that is legally enforceable. Note that New York State offers an equivalent MOLST form.

- **Do Not Intubate (DNI) Order**: This specific refusal to allow a breathing tube applies to those with *impending breathing failure* in those who are still *alive*. It seems pointless to allow CPR on someone who was in breathing distress, but no breathing tube was placed; their heart would give out anyway. Thus DNI requests make sense along with DNR (no CPR) orders. One situation in which DNI has specific importance is for those who suffer from severe lung disease like emphysema. These folks may have experienced a few bouts of intubation and intensive care unit treatment. They do not want to endure that burdensome experience again, knowing they may never get weaned off a ventilator at this advanced stage of illness. DNI makes sense for these people if they go into respiratory distress but their heart still beats. They want natural death in this situation since the breathing crisis itself means the end is near because of advanced and *irreversible* lung disease.
- **Substitute Decision Makers:** These people can be named in a Living Will but it is *not* legally binding unless Durable Power of Attorney for Healthcare or Healthcare Proxy legal forms are completed. Specific local requirements vary so search online for the details in your locale. Caveat: You are advised to choose decision makers with whom you have had discussions about your wishes and philosophies. They should understand *your* values and needs and not make decisions to "keep you around longer" based upon their own needs. Another key point: You can specify in your Living Will how much flexibility in decision-making your decision maker has. Either they must follow your instructions precisely as written in your Living Will, or they are allowed to make necessary decision adjustments based upon doctor recommendations as the

situation evolves, or the decision maker has full autonomy to make all needed decisions (this last option may be less advisable).

- **The Guilt Factor:** Most folks will find end of life decisions for loved ones painful and heart-wrenching. Many years of family dynamics, anger and hurt feelings might bubble to the surface. Even in a perfect relationship, loved ones might feel like they are hastening death if they do not treat with everything medicine has to offer. Those who are more prepared to face the dying process, and who specify with clarity and detail what their wishes are in writing, will no doubt spare loved ones much guilt, pain and anxiety during the dying process. As noted previously, research has shown that one-third of decision makers experience significant emotional effects after making end-of-life decisions, effects that may have negative impact for years. The reverse can be true as well. When loved ones put forth doubts about a dying family member's decision for end-of-life wishes, or if conflicts arise between family members it may lead to a "bad death" filled with anxiety and guilt for the sick person. Inability of loved ones to accept the dying process and death can contribute to a bad death experience. Another danger: lack of acceptance can lead to unrealistic expectations of the limits of what medicine can offer at life's end. This can result in decisions to pursue futile medical treatments that serve only to add avoidable discomfort and pain for the one who is dying. The goal is to *extend life*, not to *prolong death.*
- The media glorifies medical technology and treatments, giving folks the impression we are only a few clicks and zaps away from immortality. Not true. CPR, in fact, is rarely successful in frail older folks and only has a positive outcome in up to 15 percent of hospitalized adults of any age who suffer cardiac arrest. For old folks who choose dialysis after age 75 years, five-year survival is only 15 percent and many complications accompany the treatments. In truth, surveys have found that 75 percent of people do *not* want to die in the hospital or an ICU (intensive care unit), and there are 2.5 million people who die each year in the United States. Yet, only 37 percent of surveyed adults said they think much about end-of-life care and wishes. Let us strive to change that!

- In devising a die-happy plan, it is crucial to distinguish between reversible or treatable illness versus irreversible or terminal disease. Also, distinction should be made between illness that leads to losses that have limited negative effects versus those diseases that lead to loss of function or mental capacity and progressively weaken the body or mind, with death a direct and inevitable result.
- Planning for the end of life should be considered as a permanent retirement plan. Avoid labels and attitudinal associations of dread and fear – like doing taxes. The die-happy process should focus more on those things that bring spiritual peace and deep life meaning, not just the legalities, accounting considerations and medical procedures. If you are better prepared for the final stage of life, it will be less traumatic for yourself and loved ones. With all due respect to the poet, Dylan Thomas, I must disagree with him:

> ***Do*** go gentle into that good night... *Do* ***not*** rage, rage against the dying of the light. Though wise men at their end know dark is right.

- Live every day like it is your last. Be kind. Mend rifts. Nurture relationships. Pursue dreams and goals. Have no regrets and you will die a happy death.
- Ponder and write down your key goals and meaningful activities or accomplishments if you are diagnosed with a serious illness. These goals will serve as tonic to combat hopelessness and despair.
- Many doctors feel uncomfortable discussing end of life issues, surveys have found. If your doctor avoids the subject, or glosses over it, he or she may not give you the opportunity to deeply consider and communicate your wishes. The result: silence on the issue leads doctors to assume you want more aggressive treatments, even those therapies that offer little benefit especially at late stages of disease. For example, one study of dialysis patients found nearly two-thirds of participants regretted starting on dialysis; about half reported that their physician *chose* to initiate dialysis treatment. Speak up and start the communication process with your doctor.

Let the doctor know if you have had enough extraordinary treatments with painful side effects. It might save your *death*.

- Getting an informed prognosis for your diagnosis is surely important, but can be notoriously inaccurate and harmful. First, the same cancer type can kill someone in three months while killing somebody else in three years. Also, recall the nocebo effect: If a doctor tells you death will come soon, you might actually die sooner if you believe it to be true. Positive outlook can indeed extend life. Remaining functional capabilities and quality-of-life red lines that get crossed may be a better guide to treatment decisions and a more reliable gauge of your time left.
- If you suffer from chronic illnesses or are frail, once you have implemented a die-happy plan be sure to limit your care to one hospital, one doctor, and one active substitute decision-maker. The more cooks in your end-of-life kitchen, the greater likelihood of mucking up the recipe for a happy death. This approach can help avoid the risk someone will unknowingly not honor your final wishes due to oversight or confusion.
- Sadly, just over half of all people die in hospitals or nursing homes despite the wishes of the majority to die at home and avoid invasive procedures. Almost one-third of folks die soon after an intensive care unit admission. It is doubtful the hospital or intensive care unit is on your Bucket List of places to visit during your final weeks of life.
- **Reminder**: Any limitations or decisions you set for your "final chapter" of care can be revised at any time in the future if you have a change of heart. Perhaps new goals or life meaning have changed your mind; for instance, an upcoming grandchild's wedding that you wish to attend. Be sure to update the documents with doctors, hospitals, ambulance, substitute decision maker(s) and attorney.

Key Questions to Ask Yourself While Considering a Die-Happy Plan

- What "red lines" are there, if crossed, that would make life lose all meaning? These would make me decide I do not want my life extended. Being bedridden? Losing ability to communicate with people? Paralysis? Severe pain? Being mostly dependent on caregivers with basic daily activities? Loss of bodily function control? Loss of ability to eat real food and savor flavor and texture? Being hooked up to machines that keep you alive such as ventilator machine or dialysis? Not being able to wade in an ocean or see a sunset? Suffering from loss of memory or other higher thinking function deficits due to brain injury or dementia? Coma or persistent vegetative state?

- When you ponder death, do you consider dying to be just the final stage of life? Or do you have fears about death and dying such as pain, breathing trouble, not getting a chance to bring goals and dreams to fruition? Losing dignity? Being alone? Not saying goodbye to loved ones or missing the opportunity to mend broken relationships? Fear of what happens after death, if anything? Learning more about dying and death, reading philosophy and literature on the subject, and engaging in discussions with spiritual advisors may help alleviate some of the anxiety as you formulate your beliefs about the end of physical life.
- What accomplishments, goals or experiences make my life truly meaningful? Write down a list and begin the process of achieving those meaningful goals.
- If you were near to death or diagnosed with a terminal illness, what things would bring you the most inner peace and solace? Being with loved ones as much as possible? Travel around the world or to a location you have dreamed of visiting? Religious rituals and prayer? Spending more time in nature watching sunsets, swimming in the ocean, seeing birds build their nest? Leaving your legacy to children or grandchildren by which to be remembered? Any other wishes or important considerations for you?
- If faced with terminal or serious illness or loss of function, are there any people or larger entities to which you feel responsible? Would they give you reason to extend life? For instance, a business with employees who count on you or dependent children or a disabled loved one who needs your help. Also, can you see yourself

accepting loss of function or ambulation or chronic pain so that you could find meaning through helping others? Or perhaps creating art work or helping the poor or any other higher calling could be achieved despite your newly defined limitations?

Beware: Legal Quagmires and Clarifications

- Your Living Will becomes activated only *after* you lose your ability to make decisions, are diagnosed with legally defined terminal illness, or are in a persistent vegetative state. If you want certain care principles enforced, create your "Die Happy" plan of care and specify as much detail as possible. For instance, someone living with mild Alzheimer's disease who stipulates refusal of a feeding tube in a Living Will can have this wish overruled and receive a feeding tube. The reason: one is not technically terminally ill if one can live a few years longer, thus the feeding tube and other stated wishes in a Living Will are not yet legally in effect. An official medical order such as DNR or POLST is needed to activate your no-CPR wishes and similar extraordinary care limits while you are not actively terminally ill with a prognosis of less than 6-months to live. Without the DNR or POLST documents, paramedics and emergency room doctors will not read or honor your Living Will wish to "die naturally." "Do everything" is sadly the default setting for medical care.
- Do Not Resuscitate (DNR or DNAR) order, also known as Not For Resuscitation (NFR) in Australia, applies only AFTER the final event of breathing stoppage and/or cardiac arrest. When death arrives you will be allowed the privilege of dying naturally and no CPR will be performed. A DNR order *does not* apply to or describe any end-of- life care you wish to have in the days or months or years *prior* to that final event of heart or breathing stoppage. You should write in all specifics of major treatments wanted or refused *while still alive* onto a DNR order form, or add an attachment page signed by your doctor, so paramedics can see it and honor your wishes.
- To clarify, emergency workers must have an official doctor's order like DNR, POLST or MOLST to abide by your wishes at the end

of life. An advance Directive or Living Will is *not* legally binding to emergency medical personnel.

- If you do not define clearly your *expressed wishes*, then your health-care proxy's *substituted judgment* in making end-of-life decisions for you may be faulty. Loved ones often base murky decisions upon their own wish to keep you alive or to try everything, and to avoid guilt of accelerating your death.
- Each state in the USA or any country around the world has unique procedures and laws to follow to fulfill legal requirements of end-of-life care. Forms and required information and guidelines may be quite variable state by state for Advance Directives as well as final doctor orders for care. Check the official website for each state and country, and consider using an attorney familiar with these procedures. Search online for the state or country name followed by "advance directive form" or "do not resuscitate" to find relevant information. State Health Departments usually provide these specific laws.
- Healthcare Proxy or Surrogate obligations: Your Living Will should specify how much or how little leeway the surrogate or healthcare power of attorney has in the decision making process on your behalf, or if the proxy should simply follow to the letter your living will document and stated wishes. One-third of surrogates experience significant negative emotional effects after making a decision for an incapacitated person, and the negative effects can last for years.
- Beware of futile care, false hope, and surrogate guilt or bad intentions underlying surrogate decisions at the end of life. People still die even when hooked up to all sorts of machines and tubes. On the other hand, *realistic* hope and belief in miracles should not be abandoned. But do not let inaccurate media portrayals of CPR as being successful in 75 percent of cases mislead you. CPR is, in fact, successful in less than 15 percent of cases even while in the hospital; success rates are far lower for out-of-hospital situations and in frail, sick folks near the end of life.
- Denial in a patient or family member can swiftly turn a happy

death into an ugly mess. Sooner or later, "He can bounce back again like he's done before" no longer applies. All the tubes, machines and technology in the world will not make death optional. There comes a time when it is best to let go. A 2008 study published in *Journal of the American College of Cardiology* found that nearly one-third of patients with advanced heart failure said they would trade another two years in their current state for just one day of excellent health. A 1997 study in *Journal of the American Geriatrics Society* showed that 30 percent of seriously ill people surveyed in a hospital said they would "rather die" than live permanently in a nursing home. Clearly *quality* can be more valuable than *quantity* to many people.

- Remember that any wishes stated in a Living Will, Advance Directive, medical order or legal form such as DNR can be changed at any time. Notify all nearby hospitals and emergency rooms, local paramedics, doctors and loved ones if significant changes in last wishes are made.

DANGER 10. EMERGENCY ROOM AND HOSPITAL OVERCHARGES

Man Wakes After 12 days to a $150,000 Hospital Bill

This was the headline of a November 2013 Arizona Republic (azcentral.com) newspaper article describing Scott Richardson's ordeal. He fainted in the shower, whacked his head on tile and remained unconscious for 12 days. Why the astronomical medical bill? After all, he was insured and had been paying for Blue Cross health coverage for years. The problem: The ambulance crew transported him to Mayo Clinic hospital which was *not* contracted with his health insurance plan. With each long day he spent in intensive care, the register kept ringing up charges that were not covered. Blue Cross left him with a $120,000 bill from Mayo Clinic for which he was responsible. Richardson had to negotiate with the hospital, the insurer insisted, until media publicity convinced Blue Cross to accept responsibility for the tab. He was one of the lucky ones, and being an attorney did not hurt him either. Not everyone is so fortunate.

Scorpion Sting Leaves Ahwatukee Woman with a Big Bill

This is another shocking Arizona Republic newspaper headline from September 2012. The price tag surely stung worse than the critter: $83,000! "But how?" you might be wondering. Most Arizona scorpion stings are benign, but when the woman started to experience difficulty breathing she ended up on a hard stretcher in Chandler Regional Hospital's emergency department. This hospital, however, was out of her Humana insurance network. The two doses of antivenom for scorpion stings were billed at $39,000 each. The price in Mexico: $100 per dose, according to the azcentral.com article.

Why are healthcare costs so high?

Over one hundred years ago the federal government broke up monopolies that used their power to fix and charge high prices for needed goods and services. The oil-trust, steel-trust, sugar-trust, and railway-trust are a just few. President Teddy Roosevelt challenged those monopolies and broke them into smaller pieces, allowing for true competition. Yet 100 years later the Hospital-ER monopoly thrives without challenge. There are too many cash-paying patients and those who are insured (but out of network) who receive budget-busting bills for emergency care or hospitalization. Some folks end up in bankruptcy. The high charges for medical care in emergency departments have been characterized as shameful rip-offs. Most Americans have some type of health insurance, but it is not unusual for a health insurance company not to pay much of your emergency room or hospital bill. So why are these bills so shocking? In truth, nobody seems to know for sure, but there are clearly factors that contribute. One theory is that hospitals and emergency rooms negotiate much lower payment rates with insurers so they start with inflated and exorbitant initial prices. There is also speculation that these astronomical charges help recover costs of providing charity care to those who cannot or will not pay their bill. Some would argue that the hospital sets high prices because they have a captive group of patients like a monopoly. When challenged about overcharges, hospital executives might respond by asking, "Do you want us to close the emergency room?"

Some additional factors for high medical bills:

- It has been estimated that between 40 and 80 percent of medical bills are inaccurate, with double charges, incorrect procedures that were not performed, and unreasonable fees such as $20 per pill for a common pain killer. As another example, one hospital has charged $439 for an anti-nausea drug that costs just a few dollars.
- Unlike almost any other segment of the economy, emergency room prices are generally not posted at the entrance desk or online. You will have no idea how much the emergency visit costs until you get the bill weeks later.
- If someone is taken to an emergency room or hospital that is not contracted with the insurance carrier they have, they will end up with higher bills. Only 50 to 60 percent of reasonable and customary charges may be paid for "out of network" care, rather than the usual 80 to 100 percent of "reasonable and customary" charges that would be covered. The same holds true for individual doctor charges when that doctor is "out of network."
- An emergency room visit usually involves many different departments and services. That electrocardiogram comes with a charge for a cardiologist's interpretation. That chest x-ray will cost you a radiologist expert reading as well. Specialists called to consult will also send separate bills. Labs may well send additional bills too.
- The RAND Health Insurance Experiment (HIE), done a generation ago, found that when folks got free care they used 40 percent more services. This RAND study has become the seed for the growth of insurance co-payments and deductibles so patients get to feel the pain of cost-sharing. This approach sounds logical, however, it may cause people on tight budgets to delay seeking needed medical care early, sometimes delaying until crisis develops.
- Unnecessary tests, procedures and hospital admissions can also be a culprit. Recent lawsuits have exposed a culture of ordering useless tests and needless hospital admissions at some

emergency departments and hospitals. These unscrupulous practices stemmed from pressure on doctors to generate more income for emergency departments and hospitals, according to the publicized lawsuits.

- Fear of lawsuits leads to defensive medicine which usually involves ordering tests and treatments that offer little actual benefit. For example, an elderly woman fell at her adult care home and bumped her head. She was taken to the emergency room and found to be in good spirits with a half-dollar sized lump on top of her head. She denied feeling dizziness or head pain. She was not on blood thinners. That did not matter. She got an MRI of her brain and neck – predictably normal – before being sent back to her home. Those MRI exams could have been declined by family. Another example is when a woman hospitalized for a serious illness developed a cold sore while in the hospital. An infectious disease specialist was called in to consult on a run-in-the-mill cold sore!

The following are three actual examples of ER bills gone wild:

A middle-aged man with nausea and mild dizziness goes to an emergency room. Treatment: An anti-nausea pill. Charges on the bill: $5,000. Itemized Bill:

Doctor fees: $900

Liver blood test: $1,061

Basic Metabolic blood test: $806

CBC blood count: $391

Urine test: $139

Moderate severity ER visit, Level 3: $1,122

One bag, intravenous fluids: $490

Two commonly available pills for dizziness: $16

A 63 year-old man seeks emergency care for chest pain that might be indigestion. His wife calls an ambulance to transport him to a local ER.

After a four-hour evaluation he is sent home without a definite diagnosis for his symptoms. No medication is prescribed. His total ER bill is over $10,000! Do not forget about the $1,000 ambulance ride bill. Sure hope it was not too bumpy. Some of his itemized charges:

Doctor fees (ER physician and radiologist): $1,600

Complex care (Level 5) evaluation: $2,300

CT Scan of Chest: $4,200

Heart monitoring: $675

Intravenous line: $460

Multiple laboratory tests, some done two or three times: $1,325

Common medications (nitroglycerin and metoprolol): $375

This case might, in fact, seem like a bargain compared to a case described in the February 20, 2013 issue of Time Magazine. Author Steven Brill describes a 64 year-old woman who went to a Connecticut emergency room experiencing chest pain. She received a three-hour evaluation then was sent home with a combined ER and doctor bill of $20,000. She had no insurance.

A middle-aged woman was involved in a low-speed minor collision in California. She was able to get out of her car and describe to the police exactly what had happened. Even though she was walking around, paramedics insisted she go to the hospital to get checked out. Her emergency department evaluation took six hours and then she was released. The accident victim was given no specific treatment. Her final bill was over $30,000, not including the hefty ambulance ride charge. Her charges included:

Trauma activation charge: $12,000

Physician charges: $787

Emergency room visit evaluation: $9,200

Pharmacy - pain medications: $233

CT scan, brain $4,582

CT scan, facial bones: $2,500

CT scan, neck and cervical spine: $3,214

Note: The Trauma activation charge is billed by some, but not all, hospitals designated as level 1 or 2 trauma centers. The charge is justified by these hospitals to support the cost of a 24/7 group of doctors and nurses dedicated to trauma care. In many cases this is just a duplicate charge for services billed under different categories. Trying to get out of paying for this charge is nearly impossible.

Tips to Help Treat ER Cash-Register Pain and Anguish:

1. First and foremost, steer clear of avoidable ER visits. As described in other chapters of the book, not every problem requires emergency room services when your doctor is not quickly available. For instance, treatment by an experienced urgent care doctor is a far better option than emergency rooms for simple lacerations such as a turkey-slicing slip or glass-in-the-trash-bag laceration. Costs to repair simple finger, leg, scalp or eyebrow lacerations in an emergency room can easily come to two to three thousand dollars. Even wound glue repair can approach one thousand dollars. Complex lacerations, however, such as those that are deep or jagged, on the face, caused by power tools, or that potentially affect function like deep hand injuries or those near the eyes and lips should be managed by an experienced plastic, hand or general surgeon. They should also be treated early to limit infection risk so a trip to an emergency room may be necessary. Doctors in training should not repair these more complex injuries. Coughs, colds, ankle sprains and other minor injuries should also be managed at urgent care. Other care options to consider for minor ailments are pharmacy-based clinics, telemedicine care online, and a nurse advice hotline through your health insurer. If you stock your medicine cabinet well with first aid treatments, it can help avoid a medical visit in the future. Some over-the-counter ibuprofen can do wonders for that unexpected toothache, headache or wrenched back, for instance.
2. Call your health insurance company before an emergency ever happens. Ask them what you should do in case of a true emergency.

Confirm which of the better hospitals and emergency departments in your area are contracted with your health insurance. It is best to see it in print or online so you do not get misinformed. Notify the insurance company by telephone within 24 hours of your emergency room visit. You should keep their 24/7 phone numbers handy in your wallet. Remember to post a note on your refrigerator and keep one in your wallet listing which hospital you wish to go to if an ambulance transports you.

3. Tell the ER doctor during your initial encounter that while you are concerned about your illness, you also worry about needless risky testing and high out-of-pocket costs. If this is incorporated into the doctor's thought process early on it might save you big bucks. Do not fear politely refusing a test and asking if it can wait a couple days if you are not feeling seriously sick or are quickly improving.

4. You or an advocate should jot down any tests or treatments performed during an emergency room or hospital encounter. When your bills arrive weeks later, you may not recall which tests were actually done. Most importantly, politely decline iffy tests or treatments that may be recommended more for the doctor than the patient. For instance, an elderly woman is sent to an emergency room from a care home for confusion and low grade fever. A urinary tract infection is diagnosed, similar to her previous hospital visit two years ago. However, the ER doctor will not send her home with antibiotics until a brain MRI is done as well, even though the urine infection would explain her mental status change. The MRI, of course, showed nothing new but could lead to another few-hundred dollar out-of-pocket cost to the patient.

5. Be wary of unnecessary ER specialist consulting. If you are going to be discharged, it may be less expensive and you might get a more thorough evaluation if you see a specialist in his or her private office. Most consulting physicians have a better level of alertness and concern at 10 am rather than 3 am. It is not uncommon for specialists to be hauled in for defensive medicine and liability fear than for your absolute benefit. Extra attention can sometimes be reassuring, at other times it is useless, but it is always expensive.

6. Call the billing department and request that an itemized bill be printed and mailed to you. Hospitals routinely send out short summaries that are difficult to interpret. Check the long bill for obvious errors like tests clearly not done, double billing, tests ordered but canceled yet still on the bill, too many days of in-patient charges, and miscoding with bizarre diagnoses or procedures that have no relationship to your problem. Consider protesting outrageous charges like a $300 nausea pill that actually costs $10. They might relent. Always ask for a discount and payment plan option. Hospitals do not expect to be paid the heavily up-charged full retail price or "Gross Rate."
7. If the ER doctor wants to admit you into the hospital, confirm that you are too sick to go home and follow up with your primary care doctor within a day or two. Alternatively, perhaps intravenous therapy can begin in the emergency department and additional treatment can be continued at home or at an assisted living or nursing home ("hospital at home").
8. When a doctor or nurse hands you a prescription, always ask what it is for, whether you truly need the drug, how costly it will be, and if safer and cheaper options are possible. Also call three local pharmacies for pricing and check online prices as a guide. Huge variations in cost among pharmacies can make the extra work worthwhile. Search GoodRx.com for coupons that offer significant savings, then confirm with the listed pharmacy that they honor GoodRx coupons.
9. Consider using a "Patient Advocate" or "Medical Billing Advocate" or "Medical Billing Consultant or Specialist." Contact advocate trade organizations such as National Patient Advocate Foundation, Alliance of Professional Health Advocates, or Patient Advocate Foundation. Medical Billing Advocates of America can help you find a billing specialist company. All these companies vary in their fees from $100 per hour to a flat rate to 20 to 30 percent of the dollar amount they save you. The state of Florida takes the extra step of licensing these advocates under the Florida Division of Agent and Agency Services. Some additional

resources mentioned in a *Los Angeles Times* consumer article: advoconnection.com, healthproponent.com, claims.org.

10. Go online to check the rates other local hospitals charge for the care rendered or procedures performed on you. Use this data as comparison to determine if your bill seems outrageous. You can get this detailed information at sites such as ClearHealthCosts.com or HealthcareBlueBook.com or fairhealthconsumer.org.
11. The diagnoses that the ER doctor codes on the billing paperwork can impact whether your insurance company pays for tests, treatments and procedures. If you are taken by ambulance to an emergency room for severe chest pain and it turns out you have a bad case of gastritis, ask your ER doctor to add diagnosis codes (numbers that represent ailments) for chest pain or breathing difficulty or palpitations or other serious symptoms you had. If all the insurance company sees is "gastritis" or "acid reflux" they might refuse to pay for heart tests and procedures. The "Prudent Layperson" laws have alleviated much of this concern as it forces insurers to cover simple emergency diagnoses when a patient believed it was serious.

DANGER 11. SYNOPSIS OF EMERGENCY ROOM CARE AROUND THE GLOBE

The United States is plagued by chaotic and overcrowded emergency rooms. Overtreatment, medical errors and myriad infectious risks abound in American hospitals. These dangers pose the greatest risk for older adults, especially frail elderly. Unfortunately, the United States is no longer alone. Emergency room and hospital care has become similarly dangerous and unpredictable in Australia, Canada, United Kingdom, India (major medical centers), Germany and Israel. The result: medical errors, worse health outcomes, overtreatment and over-medication of older folks around the globe. Most people are unfamiliar with the state of emergency care around the globe. Why should you care? Older folks who live in Australia, United Kingdom, Canada and similarly affected countries can benefit greatly from the guidance in this book. As world travel among older adults continues to gain popularity, it is vital to know basic travel preparation tips and strategies to get quality medical help when sick in an unfamiliar part of the world. Your life and well being may depend upon it. What follows is a glimpse at variations in emergency care capabilities in different world regions. First, consider the following scenario:

> Kathy Curtis went airborne when a speeding moped slammed into her. The 64-year-old Ohio school teacher had crossed a potholed street in a crowded Asian city when it happened. Onlookers gathered around her while the stunned woman moaned and grimaced. Kathy's left leg was splayed out to her side and clearly deformed. A gash across her knee spurted blood, creating a red puddle in the street. A young man in the crowd removed his sweaty shirt and tried to stop the bleeding by applying pressure. Kathy was coherent enough to expect to hear the sounds of an ambulance, but no savior would ever arrive. No organized emergency medical system existed in that city.
>
> Instead, she was scooped up into the back seat of a taxi that sped off to a nearby hospital. At the entrance to the ER, the taxi driver demanded Kathy give him a $20 US greenback before he would let her out. Some men from a nearby crowd helped carry her into the emergency department, dumped her onto a gurney and pushed her into one of the overcrowded hallways. A half hour later, a nurse responded to her screams and wheeled her into a crowded exam room with six other patients. A doctor examined the wound, put a clean dressing on it and ordered an X-ray. Diagnosis: Her femur, the thigh bone, was shattered in three places. The lady was placed in a traction splint and transferred up to one of the hospital wards. Up there, an orthopedic surgeon was scheduled to see her the following day. Two days later, the orthopedist finally arrived to evaluate Kathy and had her transferred to a private hospital. Too little, too late. She had died from overwhelming infection.

Is this horror story the rule or exception in countries outside the borders of the United States? It depends, of course, on which country you are in. Emergency care in other countries runs the gamut from equal quality to America to much worse or even non-existent! Major quality differences can exist even among different regions within a single country. Prepare yourself for unpredictability and an entirely different set of rules if you live in or plan to visit a country outside the United States.

Who Should Read this Chapter?

1. You are a citizen or resident of a country outside the United States visiting another country outside of America.
2. You are a native, or long term resident of a country outside America.
3. You are a United States resident, returning to visit your native country overseas.
4. You are a United States resident who will be traveling abroad as a tourist, student or business person.

Again, emergency rooms in many countries can be terribly overcrowded. Long waits in crowded, chaotic and noisy hospitals may add to the stress of an illness or injury. This chapter offers some general guidance to help people avoid healthcare culture shock.

Different Countries, Different Rules

Forget your bad case of the runs or spiking fever. No matter that you are turning shades of yellow or blue. In some countries, you may be expected to pay when you first arrive at the facility. Alternatively, you may have to pay when you are discharged. No payment? Then risk having your passport confiscated. Exceptions exist in Europe where medical insurance may be recognized across borders. This approach contrasts sharply with the United States wherein you are mailed a bill weeks after your visit. Some United States hospitals, however, now request some payment upfront based upon your insurance copayment and deductible responsibilities.

United States Federal laws and regulations require all persons with an emergency medical condition be evaluated and get stabilizing care without regard to insurance status or available funds. Such rules do not exist in many other nations. On the bright side, paying up front may not be that painful abroad. Total care charges for simple problems might be less than 100 dollars – a bargain by American standards.

However if you need extensive treatment or get hospitalized, your bill may be hundreds, or perhaps thousands, of dollars. Hospitals and doctors abroad are unlikely to bill your insurance company: they expect upfront payment. Hospitals that cater to people from developed countries may have online web-based money transfer systems. This allows you to transfer money directly from your checking account at home. Others take credit cards. In the worst cases, your passport may be kept until you come up with the cash, so have a backup plan to get cash from friends or relatives back home.

Waiting times to see an emergency room doctor might be as short as a few minutes, and then you could be evaluated, diagnosed, treated and sent out within an hour – usually having received fine medical care. On the other side of the care spectrum, there are more than a few cases of long waits of 12 to 24 hours in overcrowded public hospitals located overseas. One group of emergency physicians in China complained that many patients got stuck in the emergency room for as long as three days!

ER Overcrowding

Public hospital emergency facilities in many countries are overcrowded, and you may wait for hours if you have anything but a serious illness or injury. Beware! Long waits in crowded emergency rooms might expose you to infections spread through the air. You should ask locals or research in advance where private hospitals are located since they may have shorter waiting times and better diagnostic and treatment facilities. In many countries, private hospitals will provide better service than public facilities. In countries that have emergency room overcrowding problems, ambulance diversions among hospitals can cause ambulances to drive in circles around a city to find an accepting hospital. Also check online with the **Joint Commission International** to see which hospitals are certified. If there are no certified hospitals, ask friends or contacts who live locally for recommendations to seek urgent care. If you will be in a specific city for an extended period, consider visiting the recommended hospitals, walking into the emergency department waiting room and asking yourself, "Would you want to be treated there?"

What are Doctor Qualifications in Overseas Emergency Rooms?

Doctor qualifications in emergency rooms abroad vary country by country. As a rule of thumb, most doctors are better trained than you might think judging by peeling paint and dilapidated conditions of some facilities in developing nations. In English-speaking countries you will most likely be treated by a fully-trained emergency care physician. In non-English-speaking country emergency rooms, a general practitioner is likely to be staffing the facility. In large teaching hospitals, several specialty emergency rooms may exist within a larger department. The medical professional performing the triage evaluation, either a doctor or a nurse, will decide which specialty area to send patients to.

Keep in mind that training requirements to become a physician differ from American requirements. English-speaking and western European nations equal or exceed United States standards. Developing nation medical care lags behind. As in America, if you go to a teaching hospital most of the doctors you encounter will be doctors in training such as interns and residents. They may try hard but lack the experience necessary for high-level care. It is advisable to then request an evaluation by the attending (senior) physician in charge.

It has taken nearly thirty years in the United States to establish Emergency Medicine as a recognized specialty. Board-certified Emergency Medicine (ER) physicians now staff most large hospitals in America. Some countries overseas have recognized the virtues of having dedicated Emergency Medicine physicians. Many countries are rapidly reorganizing emergency care, and may soon be on par with the United States standards. The International Federation for Emergency Medicine has assisted in this effort and its membership draws from emergency medicine physician societies from over 50 countries.

Preparing for Injury or Illness in Countries Other than the United States

A. First, become knowledgeable about health risk in the country you live in or plan to visit.

1. Check with the United States Centers for Disease Control and

Prevention (www.cdc.gov). The easy-to-use section on **Traveler Health** discusses health risks specific to any country and via any mode of travel from cruise ship to airplane.

2. The World Health Organization (www.who.int/en/) International Travel and Health section provides helpful information on specific countries as well as common diseases in any locality.

B. Be prepared: Get insurance.

1. If you are a United States resident, your health insurance company may not cover medical care costs delivered outside the states. Call and check with your insurer before you leave for your trip. Medicare does not cover medical care outside the United States; however, many supplemental insurance programs cover some of the costs. Find out the procedure if you submit hospital and doctor bills. Ask specifically what you need to do since the bills may be printed in a foreign language, and list foreign currency amounts.
2. Consider buying additional medical insurance coverage. At a minimum, this should include *evacuation insurance* and *supplemental travel health insurance.* Evacuation insurance will cover the costs of transporting you back to the states, if the insurance company thinks that is necessary. Don't expect to be flown back if you have pneumonia or a case of diarrhea and dehydration. Supplemental travel health insurance will provide you with a number to call to find out where you should go for emergency medical care. There are many companies that offer insurance. A web search to read reviews or complaints can be helpful. An article on the CDC website recommends using the following resources for obtaining supplemental travel and evacuation insurance: Department of State (www.travel.state.gov), International Association for Medical Assistance to Travelers (www.iamat.org), and American Association of Retired Persons (www.aarp.org).
3. If you live in a country that mandates or has government-based insurance, periodically check that your registration and health cards are up to date. If you are visiting countries beyond the borders of your country, you may need to purchase additional medical travel insurance.

C. Print in advance a list of places to go in case you have a medical emergency. Lists or recommendations of clinics or physicians who see patients any time of day can be obtained from several sources such as United States embassies or consulates and hotels. The International Society for Travel Medicine also offers lists for care in over 80 countries around the globe (www.istm.org). Print a copy to carry in your purse or wallet. Some physicians who are listed may not always see urgent cases so you will not know until you call.

1. If you live locally, ask your doctors, friends, and relatives for advice. Visit ERs in advance to gain an idea of how crowded and clean they are. Talk with hospital personnel about the training, specialty and experience of doctors who work in the hospitals.
2. *International Association for Medical Advice to Travelers* (www.iamat.org) maintains a list by country of physicians who speak English.
3. *Joint Commission International*: The US Joint Commission has reviewed standards at US hospitals for decades. An affiliated organization, the Joint Commission International conducts surveys at foreign hospitals and certifies or accredits those that meet higher standards for medical care. Not all countries have accredited hospitals, and in some countries very few hospitals achieve accreditation. For example, at press time only five of the 1,800 hospitals in Indonesia are accredited. The website www.jointcomissioninternational.org has an online list of hospitals by country, some with links to the hospital's website.
4. Buy a travel book for the country you live in or plan to visit. Some guidebooks mention clinics with addresses and phone numbers that cater to English-speaking visitors. The Lonely Planet series provides some of the greatest detail.
5. United States Embassy: Locate the United States Embassy website of the country you plan to visit by going to the central State Department embassy website. Most of these websites have information on medical care, and may list specific clinics and physicians. http://www.usembassy.gov/index.html
6. If you are an American traveler going abroad, call your health

insurance company and ask for advice. Many contract with services that can link you to English-speaking physicians and clinics. For example, health insurance companies use *Assist America*. In an emergency, hotel staff or tour guides may help you find an appropriate emergency room, clinic or hospital.

7. If you plan to be in a specific area for an extended period of time check out local hospitals. Visit their emergency facilities. Read through all the pages of their websites.

In summary: If you need a hospital, go to a Joint Commission-approved hospital if one is available. Otherwise, go to a private hospital with a good reputation. If traveling, ask hotel staff, tourist bureaus, or tour guides where travelers go for care, and who they would recommend as a local doctor. Avoid blood transfusions if at all possible. Avoid going to a foreign emergency room without a friend or advocate to keep an eye on things.

If you are traveling overseas, assemble basic and prescription medications into a travel "Sickness Sack." Ask your primary care physician for help obtaining medications you might need. Those who take prescriptions for chronic illness should bring copies of official doctor prescriptions and directions, especially for controlled substances.

Following are the key components of a "Sickness Sack" when traveling abroad:

- Diarrhea with Fever: Fever and diarrhea associated with travel to a third-world country requires immediate evaluation by a qualified medical professional. Ciprofloxacin or sulfa-based antibiotics are effective in treating severe runs with fever. Diarrhea without a fever while traveling is best treated with Azithromycin. Before leaving on a trip, ask your doctor for assistance with these prescription medications so you can be prepared. Drink plenty of fluids with salts and electrolytes if you come down with a case of the runs. Be cautious about food and water you consume while traveling abroad.
- Pain Medications: Be sure to bring along some ibuprofen or naproxen and acetaminophen for mild to moderate pain. If you

suffer from more serious chronic or episodic pain, a narcotic pain reliever should be packed. It might prevent a doctor or hospital visit abroad. Be sure to have with you copies of the doctor prescription and keep the medication in its original bottle.

- Simple pain relievers also reduce fever; however, high fever over 101 degrees might be a sign of a serious ailment picked up while traveling. A respectable ER or clinic would usually be adept at diagnosing and treating common local ailments.
- Antihistamines for Allergic Reactions: Over the counter antihistamines such as diphenhydramine, loratadine, fexofenadine or cetirizine are a vital part of a traveler "Sickness Sack" to treat allergic reactions to foods, plants, insect or animal stings or from unknown causes. Signs include itchy red rash anywhere on the body, trouble breathing, trouble swallowing, dizziness, anxiety, chest tightness or sudden wheezing, and runny nose and teary eyes. Swelling of the face, lips, tongue or neck area can also be a clue to a serious allergic reaction.
- Insect Repellants: Pack insect repellants recommended by the CDC website for travel to Malaria-endemic areas as well as places known for other insect-spread diseases. A search in the CDC site search bar will turn up valuable advice.
- Medications: Do not neglect to bring your usual medications such as inhalers for asthma, insulin for diabetes, and any necessary prescription drugs.
- Vomiting: A few anti-nausea and anti-motion sickness pills prescribed or recommended by your doctor can surely come in handy for milder bouts of puking.

ER Care by Global Location: A Summary

Following are some general observations on emergency care for specific regions of the globe. Note: Within each country emergency care can vary widely depending on the locale:

British Standard of Healthcare: Great Britain/Ireland/ Canada/ Australia/Singapore/Hong Kong/Israel and Others

Hospital ERs: In these countries, your care will likely be equal to or better than the average emergency room in America. You might well feel at home but do not get too relaxed; chaos still rules in most emergency departments so vigilance is advised. These countries follow a care model similar to that in the United States. A patient who seeks care at an ER in British-standard countries is first screened by a triage nurse who assigns a priority level. Some of these triage-scoring systems, such as the Canadian Triage System, have actually been adapted and used in the United States. If you are critically sick or injured you will rushed into the main treatment area and be promptly evaluated by a doctor. Reminder: these automated triage systems are often inaccurate in older folks (see Triage Travesty chapter).

Hospitals in British standard countries are equipped with modern diagnostic laboratories and hi-tech radiographic imaging equipment such as CT scanners and MRIs. Medications are identical or similar to those used in the United States. Blood used for transfusions has been appropriately screened for viruses. Quality of care measures are reviewed and enforced. Nurses and other professional staff are well-trained and licensed. Health care is largely government-subsidized. You may be asked to make a small payment before being treated – usually under 50 dollars.

Physicians: A patient will most likely be evaluated and treated by a specialist trained and certified in Emergency Medicine which is recognized as an important specialty. Residency training programs have set a high standard of care for these ER physicians.

ER Overcrowding: Waiting times at urban and teaching hospitals can be many hours if you are not critically ill. Expect long waits at teaching hospitals in Canada, Australia, New Zealand and urban England. These countries have actually taken the lead in publishing data on overcrowding. But that is no help to you if you are stuck waiting many hours for care. Smaller community hospitals will have shorter waiting times to see a doctor, but may lack subspecialty expertise for serious or rare diseases that teaching hospitals offer.

EMS, Trauma and Specialty Hospitals: Ambulance crews are trained to levels equivalent to United States EMTs or paramedics, with a system similar to 911. Ambulances are well stocked with equipment to stabilize emergencies and have on hand medications used in American ambulances. Good news: Medical personnel can read and react to Medic Alert bracelets. Urban areas may have specialty hospitals such as trauma and stroke centers.

Europe

Emergency Care in Western Europe is quite good. Locals who fall ill are expected to contact their primary care physician (PCP) during office hours, or call a primary care on-call doctor after office hours. Many people, however, self-refer to an emergency department for care. If you are a visitor and have no PCP you can call the local equivalent of a 911 number and be given advice on how to access urgent medical care. For example France has an advanced EMS system called SAMU (telephone is only two digits: 15, that directs you to or brings to you the type of care that matches your medical problem. In most instances the person with whom you are dealing will speak English or be able to quickly locate a translator. In Eastern Europe the situation is variable, with private hospitals in larger cities the best choice for visitors.

Hospital ERs; Most Western European emergency rooms see the sickest people first. They follow a severity-based triage system to determine the order in which patients are evaluated. The Manchester Triage System, developed in England, is used in many European emergency rooms. Hospitals are well-equipped with CTs, MRIs, modern drugs and resuscitation equipment. Hospitals must meet strict standards set in each country. Swiss emergency departments are at the top of the list for quality. Compared with Western Europe, Eastern European ERs may have less modern equipment, but generally have well-trained physicians and other staff.

Physicians: Physician quality is generally excellent but the specialty of physicians who staff these emergency rooms is variable. In many countries, Emergency Medicine is not recognized as a stand-alone medical specialty. Traditional specialties such as Surgery, Internal Medicine, or Anesthesiology provide care in the ER.

ER Overcrowding: ERs may be crowded or nearly empty, depending on the country and location. One study in Holland found that over two-thirds of the ERs were overcrowded several times each week (Derlet and co-authors). Teaching hospitals have the longest waits, private hospitals the shortest waits. In Urban areas expect to wait if you have a minor problem. If you are a local resident, ask your doctor or friends about the best hospitals before crisis strikes.

EMS: A central number similar to 911 dispatches Ambulances. Some countries, such as France and others, have a two-tier system; a basic Paramedic response ambulance or an advanced Physician response ambulance. Yes, a *doctor* is part of the ambulance team for more severe emergencies and comes with a fully stocked ambulance, like a mini "ER on wheels."

Latin America

Hospital ERs from Mexico south to the tip of Argentina can fall into one of many categories, even in the same city: (1) Government general hospital ER (2) Government- operated teaching hospital ER (3) Private hospital ER (4) Police or military hospitals with an emergency department. If you live in Latin America, do some advance planning and learn in advance the hospitals that provide better ER care. If you are visiting, don't expect everyone to speak English. Bring a language book that has a medical section so you can point to key words or phrases. If you have a smart phone with web access you can get key phrases translated through several sites that can be found on search engines.

ER Overcrowding: Public hospitals in urban areas are quite overcrowded so expect long waits. Private hospital ERs are the least crowded, and provide the best care, but expect payment in advance to the tune of hundreds, or perhaps thousands, of dollars. Diagnostic lab tests and radiology imaging services are better at private hospitals but may not always meet American standards of lowest possible dose radiation exposure. Rural area hospitals might have only rudimentary ability to care for serious emergencies. Remote areas such as the Amazon may be hundreds of miles away from medical facilities and only accessible by air or boat.

Physicians: Most Latin countries now have professional ER societies with the goal of standardizing emergency care within each country. This includes the training of physicians in emergency medicine as well as demanding that hospitals modernize their facilities. Board-certified emergency physicians are usually found only in big cities, at the teaching hospitals, where waits are long. At private or smaller community hospitals expect to be seen by a general surgeon, general practitioner or Internist. The quality of care you receive will depend on that doctor's training and experience.

EMS: Variable. Multiple types of ambulance services can exist side by side: private, civil service, public, or police. Most urban areas have organized ambulance services with a central dispatcher. Rural areas may not have organized ambulance services.

Africa

If you are a visitor to or resident of a country in Africa I strongly recommend you plan in advance for an emergency. Learn which hospitals are best. Friends, relatives, local residents, local physicians, Hotels and embassies can help guide you. Private hospitals are more likely to provide care similar to western countries. South Africa has the largest number of hospitals with modern emergency rooms that resemble a western model. Public hospitals can be terribly overcrowded and require long waits for less serious care. Egypt and its Mediterranean neighbors are similar, although standards of care in rural areas may be much lower.

If you venture off the well-beaten tourist paths into less developed sub-Saharan areas you may be in for a shock. Hospitals are frequently overcrowded, chaotic and lacking in the sanitary standards you may be accustomed to. They might have limited testing and treatment capabilities. Rural area hospitals may not even have a formal emergency room, instead providing a clinic during business hours and an admitting area for nighttime emergencies. The after-hours admitting area will only have a nurse present for illness screening purposes. She will then have to summon a physician, if needed. Many smaller towns and villages may not have a hospital, just a clinic.

A traditional practice known to many areas involves pharmaceuticals. The hospital physician will direct a relative of a sick patient to buy needed medicines at a neighboring pharmacy, and bring it back to the hospital to be administered. Patients admitted for inpatient care will have to pay extra for meals or arrange for someone to bring them food. Private hospitals, where they can be found, generally offer a better standard of care.

Physicians: Most physicians on the continent are not trained in Emergency Medicine. The African Federation for Emergency Medicine has over ten member countries at the time of press. A major goal of the organization is to implement a uniform standard of care among physicians in African emergency rooms.

EMS: Highly variable. In South Africa and Mediterranean countries formal ambulance services exist in the urban areas. Rural areas of sub-Saharan Africa are usually without modern emergency medical ambulance systems.

Asia

Emergency rooms in some countries such as Japan, Taiwan and Korea, are modern and provide care on the same level as English-speaking countries. In less developed countries, for example Bangladesh and Laos, hospital ERs may provide just rudimentary care. Private hospitals in India may provide excellent care, whereas public hospitals may not have the standards you expect. Wide variability in the quality of care occurs in the world's most populous country, China. Private hospitals in urban areas may offer care equal to western standards. Teaching hospitals have variable quality and are usually crowded. Government-run urban and rural hospitals provide basic emergency stabilization. Hospitals in certain countries may rotate in a coordinated fashion what days they accept emergency cases.

Hospital ERs: As a rule of thumb, public hospitals may be crowded and substandard. The waits for care, even if you are critically ill or injured may be long. This is what happened in the tragic case described at the beginning of the chapter. On the other hand, many private hospitals in Asia provide high quality care. Ask people in the medical field, embassy staff or locals which hospitals provide the best care and where tourists and local business people and politicians go for care. Some hospitals in Asia have standards equal to America. Some people fly from the United States to undergo elective surgeries such as hip replacements in certain Asian hospitals.

Physicians: In most nations formal recognition of Emergency Medicine as a separate specialty has not yet occurred and care is provided by surgeons or internists. However many nation-based Emergency Medicine Physician Associations have been founded over the past decade. Similar to other regions of the globe, their missions include implementation of a uniform standard of emergency care and modernizing emergency rooms.

EMS: Fire-based EMS systems provide ambulance and first-responder services in the more developed countries. Most of these systems are single-tiered, with ambulances equipped for basic life support only. Korea, Japan, Singapore, and Bangkok have intermediate emergency medical technician (EMT) service levels, while Taiwan has more advanced paramedic services. India, Pakistan and some other nations may not have organized EMS systems in every city. Rural areas commonly lack these systems. In some towns and cities no "emergency" ambulances exist, instead, one calls a taxi or flags down a motorist if emergency transport to a hospital is needed.

SECTION V.
KEY SYMPTOMS AND SIGNS YOU SHOULD KNOW ABOUT

I. ABDOMINAL PAIN: ENIGMA WRAPPED INSIDE A RIDDLE

Three older folks are on stretchers in their respective emergency departments. What do these three patients have in common?

1. An elderly woman crochets while sitting up on the stretcher. Her complaint is abdominal discomfort and constipation.
2. A frail older man with dementia has stopped eating, acts confused and swings his arms at anyone who touches him.
3. An active 80-year-old gentleman complains of on-and-off abdominal discomfort for several weeks as he went about his usual busy routine.

The answer: They all had life-threatening ruptured appendicitis. People of any age can have unusual manifestations of disease, but seniors commonly do not show the usual signs and symptoms of serious illness. Fever, severe pain, elevated white blood cell count, and rock-hard abdomen from involuntary tensing of muscles are some signs and symptoms that are frequently absent in older adults who suffer from serious abdominal ailments. What's more, twenty percent of older adults who have appendicitis seek help after three days of symptoms, and another 5-10 percent after one week of symptoms. This abdominal emergency proves deadly in ten times more older adults than in the younger crowd.

Abdominal Pain: The Red Flags

More than one in 20 visits to emergency departments are for abdominal pain complaints. So is your belly discomfort just gas pain from eating chili? Irritable bowel? Or a ruptured appendix? The cause for abdominal pain can be minor or life-threatening. Surprisingly, the diagnosis often remains unknown after an emergency room visit. Following are some clues to consider that make any abdominal discomfort *more* likely to be serious. If any or several of these red flags are present your abdominal pain is *more* likely to be a true emergency. It is then wise to seek medical care quickly either at your trusted doctor's office, a reliable urgent care facility, or an emergency department, depending upon the severity.

▶ Age: Chances go way up that abdominal pain has an ominous cause in folks over age 50.

▶ Pain Intensity: Worst-ever or intolerable pain in the gut? Cannot do even the simplest of tasks due to pain? Get checked at an emergency room promptly! For tolerable belly pain that may or may not stop your routine get checked promptly at urgent care or your family doctor if it persists more than a few hours. Nuisance pains that come and go might be familiar to you such as a urinary tract infection, true heartburn (not angina-type heartburn) or gas pains. Consider trying simple treatments such as antacids for *familiar* "indigestion", anti-gas tablets for gas pains and so on. One caveat: The elderly have reduced pain perception so pain intensity is less reliable. Each person, of course, has his or her own pain tolerance.

▶ Pain Patterns:

a. *Perpetual Movement Versus Still as a Statue* – If abdominal pain forces you to remain still as a statue and causes agony with movement, that could be a sign of inflammation and infection inside your abdomen (peritonitis). If the pain has you writhing around like a fidgety toddler or pacing the room like a father-in-waiting, this pain pattern also suggests more ominous underlying disease such as kidney stones. Get to an emergency room immediately for any of these severe pain responses.

b. *Fast and Furious Versus Waves on a Beach* – Sudden, severe, constant pain that does not much release its grip is a key red flag that should send you racing to an ER. If pain comes and goes like waves on a beach and is tolerable, it is less likely to be immediately life-threatening so you can try simple remedies and get an appointment with your doctor within a couple of days. The exception: Fever or persistent vomiting along with the pain which requires immediate attention.

▶ Fever: It is always wise to check your temperature with a reliable thermometer if you experience abdominal pain. If your temperature is over 100 degrees Fahrenheit it makes the situation dicier. Sorry, but rectal temperature tends to be more accurate.

▶ Vomiting: Nausea and vomiting (N/V) are perhaps the most feared accompanying symptoms when you suffer from abdominal discomfort. The N-V one-two punch can, if nothing else, cause misery and quickly lead to dehydration. This combination also makes abdominal discomfort more likely to be serious with diagnoses such as gallbladder disease, heart disease, kidney stones or simply a bad case of stomach virus or food poisoning. Sudden loss of appetite alone can be the equivalent of the N/V combination in frail elders.

▶ Diarrhea: The runs can also cause dehydration quickly, particularly in folks with other chronic ailments. This sign is also worrisome for those experiencing abdominal discomfort.

▶ Blood: Do you see red? In fact, blood comes in different varieties. First, black, tarry, smelly *poop*; Second, coffee ground (dark brown-black) or bright red *vomit*; and lastly, maroon or bright red *stool*. Notice any of these shades of intestinal disease and you should seek medical advice immediately, especially if it happens more than once. Note: Bright-red is most feared. Needless to say, a one-time red blotch on toilet paper is not as concerning as multiple bowel movements with red blood or clots in the toilet bowl. The caveat: Beets, blueberries, Pepto Bismol (bismuth salicylate) and iron supplements can falsely mimic these color shades of blood. Pay attention to what you ingest and it might help avoid a wasted ER visit.

▶ Risky Medications: Certain medications create greater risk for serious abdominal problems such as ulcers, bleeding or liver injury. The most notorious of these medications are aspirin, ibuprofen, naproxen, prednisone and "statin" drugs for elevated cholesterol. Alcohol use can also be toxic to the liver or stomach. Needless to say, any medication or pill can cause stomach upset and should be stopped if abdominal discomfort develops. A family doctor visit might be prudent.

▶ Back pain: Diseased abdominal organs can cause back pain as well. Examples include kidney stones or infection (flank pain), gallstones or infection (mid to upper back pain), artery tears, ovary or testicular diseases, and pancreas inflammation to name a few. Unfamiliar back pain that is not clearly aggravated by bending or twisting movements can be the equivalent of abdominal pain or angina (chest pain). Do not quickly dismiss as a pulled muscle any unfamiliar or severe back pain, especially when it occurs along with discomfort or other symptoms in the abdomen or chest region.

▶ Upper Abdominal or Chest Discomfort: Heart attacks can cause sufferers to perceive abdominal rather than chest symptoms. What's more, sometimes heart attack pain is described as "indigestion." A golden rule for patients and doctors: Think chest problems with abdominal pains and think abdominal problems in someone suffering from chest discomfort. Never separate these two body cavities despite the diaphragm muscle anatomically dividing them (see also, Chest Pain chapter). That said, about one-third to one-half of seniors have gallstones, making this diagnosis quite common in those with pain high in the abdomen or lower chest.

▶ Rapid Heartbeat or Low Blood Pressure: Fever, bleeding, dehydration, and inflammation/infection can cause a rapid heart rate (over 100 beats per minute) to develop in someone with abdominal pain. Low blood pressure (under 100 mm Hg, top number) can result from serious infection, bleeding or dehydration. These changes in vital signs are worrisome and require emergency medical evaluation. Remember: consider a person's baseline or usual heart rate or blood pressure for comparison. Caveat: Many seniors take medication that slows the heart rate thereby nullifying rapid heart rate as an early sign of serious disease. The solution can be to know that person's baseline heart rate so a significant increase from 60 to 82 beats per minute can be a key clue.

What to Expect in the Emergency Department?

If red flags are present with your abdominal pain, seek care at the hospital emergency room. What can you expect the process of care to be? Read on for greater clarity.

- **Triage** – Don't let emergency department (ED) staff keep you in the waiting room. Abdominal pain in older adults should always be considered an emergency priority until proven not to be serious! Speak up and ask for the doctor to triage you if your bad abdominal pain is being ignored or minimized. Your life might depend upon it! Ambulance transport will get you into the main ED quickly but can cost hundreds of dollars out of pocket. It is concerning that most triage software systems used in the emergency room ranks abdominal pain only in the middle of five levels of urgency (see also, Triage Travesty).
- **Nurse and Provider** (doctor, nurse practitioner, physician assistant, student, doctor-in-training) **Encounters** – At the least, a quick medical history and focused exam should be done. They might choose to start intravenous fluids if you appear weak or dehydrated or are vomiting. Blood tests and urinalysis will often be sent to the lab. Pain or nausea medication for comfort should be offered early on. If not, request it if you are truly uncomfortable. An electrocardiogram should be routinely done in adults. The provider might order specialized imaging such as ultrasound, CT scan or MRI.
- **Imaging** – KISS rule applies here: ***Keep it simple & safe*** initially then move on to riskier tests (or treatments) if no answers are found. Your treating provider should discuss the benefits and risks of any tests ordered, as well as all testing and treatment options that might be helpful.
- **Observation** – Time and intravenous fluids cure many maladies so it is commonplace to be observed in the emergency department while fluids drip into your vein. By the time all tests are done and results get back to the doctor or other provider, one or two bags of intravenous fluid will likely make you feel much better, as will the medication given. If not feeling much improved, there is a good

chance your ailment is more serious and requires additional treatment, surgery or just observation in the hospital.

- **Treatments** – The primary job of the emergency room doctor is to assume your belly pain is life-threatening and dangerous. This should be the golden rule in people over age forty-five. Severe pain in the abdomen will either improve with intravenous fluids and some time or deteriorate quickly. If it is unrelenting then surgery might be the only treatment. If imaging tests rule out life-threatening illness then the focus shifts to giving intravenous fluids for dehydration, pain and nausea medication as needed for comfort, observation for several hours, and correcting electrolyte imbalances like low potassium or sodium. Oftentimes these simple measures lead to marked improvement in several hours whether or not a specific diagnosis is pinpointed.
- **Specialist Consultation** – A specialist should be called in to evaluate you for several reasons:
    1. If you are vomiting or pooping blood then a gastroenterologist might need to "scope" you and look inside your stomach or large intestine to find the source of bleeding.
    2. If there is concern about appendicitis or a rupture or hole in your intestine or stomach or a tear in a blood vessel or some other catastrophic organ disease in your abdomen or pelvis. In any of these scenarios a surgeon or gynecologist will be consulted.
    3. If your abdominal discomfort proves to be a heart problem, based upon an electrocardiogram and special blood tests, then a cardiologist might be called in.
    4. If it remains unclear to the provider and emergency room physician-in-chief what is making you sick, then you should request a second opinion from a specialist if simple treatments mentioned above have not worked.
- **To Admit or to Discharge** – The decision whether to bring you into the hospital or send you home is simple. If intravenous fluids and simple treatments have made you feel much better, and lab

tests and imaging studies do not find anything serious, discharge home is appropriate. *Beware*! It is critical to follow up within a day or two with your family doctor or return to the ER if problems persist or deteriorate. Sometimes serious disease is masked in the early stages and tests cannot find the problem at this initial stage of illness. When your condition is persistent or deteriorating, do not assume all is okay since the ER did not find anything wrong initially.

Appendicitis Tips

Since half of all appendicitis deaths occur in older adults, some tips and pearls are worth mentioning and are relevant for all types of serious abdominal disease in older folks.

The longer the delay in diagnosis of significant abdominal pain the greater the chances for complications such as perforation (rupture), pus pockets, blood infection, and death. Paradoxically, older folks tend to delay seeking medical care longer than younger adults. Once they do get help, the *initial* diagnosis proves incorrect up to 50 percent of the time in appendicitis cases. What's more, older folks have reduced ability to compensate because of other ailments such as heart disease and diabetes. It's a triple whammy! An inflamed appendix will typically rupture within 48 hours. Patient delays seeking care and diagnosis delays in the emergency department add up to misdiagnosis and possible complications.

What is the textbook description of appendicitis that is typical in younger adults? First, there is sudden onset of vague abdominal pain usually around or above the belly button. Next comes loss of appetite, nausea or vomiting. Third in line will be low grade fever. Within hours a sharp and more severe pain will localize in the right, lower belly as the lining of the abdominal cavity gets inflamed near the appendix. Constipation is far more common than diarrhea.

In older and frail adults, all bets are off. Throw the textbook away since less than one-third of older folks show the classic signs of appendicitis. Amazingly, nearly one-third of older folks seek care between three and seven days after symptoms began! There are several unique challenges to determining just how serious pain in the abdomen is in older and ***frail*** adults:

- Grandma will often be vague and say she's just feeling weak. Dementia, stroke or hearing impairment may further complicate communication difficulty. Loss of appetite or loss of functional ability such as not walking anymore might be the only clue a frail senior is ill.
- The elderly tend to look less sick even when seriously ill. They are less sensitive to pain and are less likely to spike a fever. Younger adults will develop a hard, "board-like" abdomen with peritonitis as their belly muscles reflexively tense up when pressed; this finding is usually absent in seniors. The all important elevated white blood cell count typical in younger adults is also less frequently present in older sufferers. In fact, lower right-sided belly pain, fever and elevated white blood cell count are *all* present in only *one-quarter* of folks over age 60 years. This explains why doctors too commonly misdiagnose serious abdominal illness in older folks.
- Seniors tend to delay seeking help for sudden illness for reasons such as fear of going to the hospital, fear of death, concern over the cost of medical care, or simply not wanting to bother anybody. One published case report, as mentioned earlier, describes an elderly woman suffering from abdominal discomfort and constipation who was crocheting on the stretcher in the emergency department as her appendix was rupturing! A CT scan clinched the diagnosis.
- The odds are stacked against older adults since they are more likely to require hospital admission and surgery for a complaint of abdominal pain. One-half to two-thirds of seniors with abdominal pain in the ER will require hospital admission. One-third will require surgery. Even with fancy technology, up to 30 to 40 percent of older folks will not get a definite diagnosis for their belly pain – testimony to the limitations of tests and technology.
- Never let an older adult with abdominal pain get discharged from the ER unless they are feeling much better. *Reminder*: Many serious abdominal illnesses begin with tolerable symptoms that seem

minor, particularly in older adults who have reduced pain perception. The emergency room doctor's job is to exclude serious causes (including chest problems like heart attack) before considering discharge home.

- Seniors take medications that can predispose them to abdominal ailments. For instance, pain relievers and prednisone.
- Older folks have reduced ability to fight infection; they also suffer from ailments such as heart disease or diabetes. These health problems limit their ability to compensate for the body stress of serious abdominal disease. As mentioned, one-half of all deaths from appendicitis occur in those over age 60 years. What's more, the appendix ruptures in 30 to 70 percent of older adults with this ailment, a much higher rate than in their younger counterparts.

Visceral Pain: First Clue to Serious Organ Disease

When an organ in the chest, abdomen or pelvis suddenly becomes starved of enough blood, stretches or gets inflamed it triggers *visceral* pain. This pain is felt as a vague, deep discomfort around the center or midline of the body. Prime examples include the breastbone area during a heart attack or the belly button vicinity with appendicitis. This type of pain is almost always accompanied by reflexive nerve responses such as profuse sweating, nausea, vomiting, racing heart, pale skin color, and a feeling of impending doom or anxiety. This early pattern of pain can be typical of any serious organ disease, not just appendicitis and heart attack. As the lining around the diseased organ gets inflamed, the pain quality changes to sharp with an easily defined location (lower, right abdomen for appendicitis, for instance). The sharper, localized pain is called *somatic* pain. Knowing these pain patterns can be helpful in identifying when discomfort or pain might be serious, requiring prompt medical care.

Some Final Key Tips:

a. Tests give clues to a diagnosis but are imperfect. Never assume a "normal" test means all is okay even if you continue to feel quite ill.

b. People suffering from serious abdominal or pelvic inflammation or infection tend to remain still and on their side, curled at the waist with knees pulled in closer to the chest. Riding over bumps while in the car aggravates the pain as does coughing or sneezing.

c. It is not unusual for appendicitis sufferers to experience urinary symptoms and have mildly abnormal urine tests. Do not let your ER provider jump to an incorrect diagnosis of "urinary tract infection" based upon a slightly abnormal urinalysis. Urine screening tests are often inaccurate or misinterpreted in older adults who are sick in the emergency room.

d. There are three simple tests anyone can perform which suggest abdominal pain is more serious:

   1. *Heel-Drop*: Stand on your toes for ten seconds then come down with all your weight on your heels. Significant pain felt in the abdomen is concerning.

   2. *Cough Test*: If coughing intensifies abdominal pain it is worrisome.

   3. *Hopping on One Foot*: If you can do this while your belly throbs without any problems, you have far less cause for concern. If you can do this at all, in fact, then you are in pretty good shape. If the belly pain jolts you while hopping then seek medical care promptly.

d. Risk factors for perilous abdominal disease include dementia, cancer, kidney failure, diabetes, HIV, alcohol abuse and taking medications such as aspirin, narcotic pain relievers or prednisone.

e. If sent home, you must get quick follow up in one or two days if symptoms are not fully resolved. Be sure you can get in to see your primary care doctor or a specialist. *Caveat*: It is never prudent to accept medical care over the telephone for serious complaints such as abdominal pain. If your doctor does not feel any urgency to see you for this problem then find another doctor immediately or seek urgent care.

f. Never leave the ER if you hardly feel better compared to when you arrived. Ask for a second opinion from a specialist if the ER doctor wants to send you home while still feeling quite ill and without getting any answers.

g. Do not forget the chest! Chest problems can manifest as abdominal pain or other intestinal symptoms.

h. Whether or not you seek medical care for abdominal distress, it is prudent to switch for a couple of days to a bland diet and soft foods like yogurt, bananas, toast, rice and chicken broth (to name a few suitable foods). Avoid sweets, spicy, caffeine and carbonated drinks. Consider ginger root and herbal tea. Hold off on any non-essential pills you take.

II. IDENTIFYING CHEST PAIN AND HEART DISEASE: TIME FOR A NEW APPROACH

Chest pain diagnosis can confuse even the brightest doctors. A doctor-in-training once asked an experienced cardiologist to predict the result of a heart angiogram being performed on a middle-aged woman. Her unusual chest pain symptoms were quite different from textbook heart attack descriptions. The young doctor grinned as he challenged the cardiologist to admit the angiogram would be normal.

"Clearly the woman's symptoms were inconsistent with heart disease pain," the novice doctor insisted.

"The only thing I know for sure," the cardiologist answered with Confucius-like wisdom, "is that I can *never* know for sure."

Consider the following three actual anecdotes that shed further light on the enigmatic nature of heart disease and its hallmark sign – chest area discomfort:

A young mother brushes off the indigestion and fatigue she has experienced for a few weeks, attributing the symptoms to her recent delivery. One morning she awakens her husband to tell him she is not feeling well. She suddenly turns blue and passes away. Chest compressions could not bring her back. An autopsy found she was born with abnormal heart-feeding arteries. She was metaphorically a ticking time bomb that might have been set off by the stress of her recent pregnancy and delivery. Nobody could have known the significance of the vague "indigestion" in her chest or upper abdominal area and the seemingly innocent fatigue symptoms.

*

An elderly woman experiences sudden "chest pains" and is rushed to a nearby hospital. Doctors order an electrocardiogram and nuclear stress test since they suspect a heart condition. The results: No indication a heart condition caused the chest pain symptoms. She is sent home but returns a few days later suffering from abdominal pain and vomiting. Ultimately, the woman has her stone-filled gallbladder removed and the chest symptoms resolve.

*

A 35-year-old man dials 911 when his sudden chest pain becomes unbearable. He tells emergency room doctors he feels dizzy and is having breathing difficulty. His chest x- ray and electrocardiogram show subtle abnormalities but are inconclusive. Likely because he is so young, he is sent home with the diagnosis of "viral illness," which actually means doctors have no clue what is wrong. He is rushed to a different emergency room two days later with the same severe chest discomfort. Diagnosis: Virus. Disposition: Sent home again… this time, to die. He was found dead on his kitchen floor, just about the same day that the musical "Rent" first opened in New York City to rave reviews. The man's name was Jonathan Larson and he was the hit musical's creator. Mr. Larson never made it to enjoy opening night. His ultimate diagnosis: A ruptured aortic aneurysm, which is a tearing of a ballooned and weakened artery such as the Aorta, the major blood-carrying tube that feeds the entire body.

*

It is estimated that between 8 and 10 million people each year rush to emergency rooms across the United States with a complaint of "chest pain." Millions more seek similar care across the globe. Diagnosing the cause for "chest pain" is *never* easy, contrary to popular perception. Consider this: Six people describe experiencing chest discomfort or pain. The first undergoes the heart procedure angioplasty to treat an artery blockage. The second person improves over several days with better diet and antacid medication. The third person takes a sedative to extinguish the symptoms, and the fourth uses the pain reliever ibuprofen to find relief. The fifth sufferer gets an antibiotic and feels much better in a few days. The last chest pain sufferer undergoes surgery to remove a diseased gallbladder and soon heals. Each of these people had somewhat different descriptions of the type of discomfort or pain they experienced, but many overlapping features were present. The reason for the confusion is that many different body organs can send or refer pain signals to the chest region including the heart, lungs, stomach and other digestive organs, ribs, chest muscles, chest arteries and even the brain. Every cause of chest pain can have unique features, but sufferers tend to be vague and inconsistent in how they describe their own experience of chest discomfort. My dull ache might be your sharp, crushing pain. Moreover, it is not unusual for a heart attack sufferer to describe chest symptoms as pressure or indigestion, for instance. People often tell doctors, when asked, that the sensation in the chest is *not* pain. To confuse the diagnosis even further, up to one-third of heart attack sufferers do not experience *any* definite chest discomfort, particularly so for the elderly, women and diabetics.

So what are the key factors doctors consider when making a diagnosis of heart disease? First, what other symptoms are present with the chest area discomfort such as heart-pounding, breathing trouble, nausea and vomiting, weakness or dizziness, profuse sweating, feeling impending doom or ghost-like pale appearance. Pain or discomfort might travel to other areas such as the mid-back, shoulders, neck, arms or jaw. As mentioned above, the description of the chest symptoms can be helpful but misleading. Heart attack sufferers have described chest pain as sharp, severe, crushing, dull, hot feeling, pressure, someone sitting on my chest, constricting, an ache, heartburn, and many other adjectives. Second, how sick the patient appears is a key factor, and if vital signs like heart rate and blood pressure are abnormal. Third, does the patient have risk factors for heart disease (see risk factors below)? Fourth, do test results such as blood tests, x-rays, or electrocardiogram show minor or obvious abnormalities? Lastly, does the patient improve with the treatment used based upon the presumed diagnosis. For example, is ibuprofen clearly helping the man's chest pain that developed soon after lifting heavy weight? If so, the chest pain more likely is caused by a pulled muscle.

Time is Muscle: Don't Be a Denier, Worrier, Procrastinator

Pick your cliché: "You snooze, you lose." "Early bird gets the worm." Clearly, arriving late to the party is not always fashionable. The major cause for delays in getting heart-muscle-saving treatment for heart attack is sufferer delay in seeking medical care. The goal is to get heart attack sufferers needed treatment within the critical one to two hours after symptoms begin when clot-dissolving treatments are most effective at reversing or limiting heart damage. Patient delays in seeking medical care are common, however, and have been well-described in the United States, Australia, Britain and Canada.

Patient Delays in Seeking Care for Chest Discomfort

So let us drill down to the root of this devastating delay dilemma which has not improved through two decades of public health campaigns on heart disease. Why do chest discomfort sufferers frequently delay for hours before seeking care when stricken with a potentially serious, but treatable, disease? The answer: It's complicated. Many factors contribute to patient delays in seeking immediate care:

1. **Denial** that one is very ill is a key delay factor. When crisis strikes, people try to minimize its severity as a defense and coping mechanism. With serious illness, we minimize the symptom experience, might self-diagnose and try to explain it away as a minor problem, or we may pepper circumstances with magical thinking. We tend to wait, wishing for scary symptoms to just go away. After all, we are too busy to be sick. When something truly bad happens, we sometimes ignore the obvious. We refuse to believe our lyin' eyes. We try desperately to continue our normal routine. Call it the Ostrich Effect – sticking one's head in the sand. "Analysis paralysis" or "wearing blinders" are other popular terms that apply. But it is real. A surge of adrenaline during crisis situations can fog the mind; in movies, that epinephrine rush leads to trembling, sweaty hands that causes a woman to drop her car keys as an attacker approaches; and it also blurs or constricts vision. Effectiveness of action drops precipitously. It may even be hard to find the phone and dial 911.

One particularly effective but dangerous form of denial is for sufferers to assign more palatable diagnoses to their symptoms. Stick any label on it. Indigestion, pulled muscle, stress or gallbladder attack are a few favorites. These labels then remove the urgency from sudden sickness since indigestion or stress are quite benign and improve with time. Inaction becomes a "reasonable" option based upon false self-diagnosis. A nap sounds good. Perhaps call friends, family members or the family doctor for opinions? All this delay allows precious heart muscle to die. Calling the family doctor, in this case, can waste precious time since he or she will simply tell you to go to an emergency room to get checked out. The exception: asking your family doctor or an educated or clear-thinking friend or relative for advice can be helpful in reorienting the sufferer to the possibly serious nature of the situation.

2. **Psychological Barriers — 50 Ways to Avoid Getting Help**: "I don't want to bother anybody." "I am too busy to be sick today." "I've got to get to work." "I must drive the kids to soccer practice soon." "Maybe I will just take a nap until symptoms go away." "What will the nosy neighbors think if I call an ambulance? The flashing lights will make a scene." "I don't want to make a fuss over nothing and waste everyone's time." "It's late at night. I will wait until morning to see if I feel better." "I'm way too young to be having a heart problem." "I exercise. Only fat, old men get heart attacks." "Without real chest pain this must just be indigestion. Get the antacids." Think of some other excuses you have heard or yourself used in past experiences.

3. **Lack of Information**: Many heart attack sufferers show shock that their symptoms were, in fact, a heart problem. Perhaps they were unfamiliar with less typical symptoms of heart disease and their personal risk factors. The Hollywood image of heart attack occurs less commonly and can be misleading. People who experienced less typical heart attack symptoms took more than six hours to seek medical care, considerably more time than those who had textbook or classic symptoms, according to studies. In fact, those who have atypical symptoms of a heart attack are more likely to be misdiagnosed. Knowledge not only can empower patients, but can

help people educate their doctors and avoid misdiagnosis in busy offices or chaotic emergency rooms.

4. **Need to Remain in Control**: Some people by virtue of their personality must always stay in control of a situation, even to their own peril. They will not surrender to the crushing sensation in the chest – no way. The labored breathing – no big deal. Nausea and profuse sweating – I can take it. Feeling faint – give me more! If they do give in and consider getting help, they will do it their own way and in their own time. Meanwhile, heart muscle might be dying off and a serious heart rhythm irregularity can end it all if the attack is bad enough. Be aware of this trait if you have it. The trait can serve you well at other times, just not when sudden and serious illness strikes.

5. **Elderly**: Older folks have additional obstacles to seeking prompt care when suffering a heart attack. They are more likely to experience less typical major symptoms such as fatigue or weakness, or loss of a daily function they could perform prior. Difficulty breathing, vomiting, confusion or simply "not feeling well" are common complaints. The elderly tend to have less chest pain, in part because they are less active, and activity is what sparks angina chest pains. Seniors may lack social support so may not have anybody available to ask for help. They might be reluctant to ask a caregiver for assistance out of fear of inconveniencing the person. Older folks may also suffer from memory loss or other communication-limiting ailments such as aphasia due to stroke or hearing impairment. There is also some evidence the elderly might have reduced pain sensation leading to understating how ill they truly are. What's more, older adults often fear dying at the hospital or never returning to their home. Additionally, the diagnosis of heart attack is murkier in the elderly because older folks might have an already abnormal electrocardiogram, as well as many other illnesses that can complicate the picture. For instance, they might surmise that known emphysema is causing the breathing difficulty and ignore the developing heart attack.

Key Tips that May Save Your Life: Brand New Approach

- No More **Pain**! Many folks perceive heart attack symptoms as *not* being pain. Any *significant* and *unfamiliar* **discomfort** – pressure, sharp, crushing, hot feeling, burning, indigestion, cramp, bubble – should prompt seeking immediate **emergency room** care.
- No More **Chest**! Think '**Chabdomen**' instead, meaning unusual discomfort from chin to chest down to belly button (chin to chest to abdomen). Adding in other 'grouped symptoms' multiplies the concern as explained below. Locations for heart attack discomfort differ in each individual as mid-back discomfort near the shoulder blades can be the primary location of discomfort (think *back* and '*chabdomen*'). Incredibly, some folks have just suffered a severe headache and vomiting as the presentation of their heart attack! In addition, recall the abdomen-chest connection. Abdominal symptoms can reflect a problem in the chest. Chest symptoms can be caused by abdominal ailments.
- **Grouped Symptoms** that come on together is a major red flag for heart attack. These symptoms can include nausea, vomiting, diarrhea, soaking sweats, heart pounding, trouble breathing, unusual anxiety or feeling of impending doom, ghost-like pale appearance, and dizziness. When should you suspect the worst? Shoulder joint pain is not usually connected to nausea and vomiting, for instance. True heartburn is not typically connected with labored breathing or dizziness. Pains in an arm from a pinched neck nerve should not come on with a racing heart.
- Any doctor making a snap diagnosis based on assumptions and attitudes is often incorrect. Any doctor or healthcare provider who is dismissive of the *possibility* of heart disease in somebody with unusual symptoms in the back or 'chabdominal' area is either inexperienced or foolish. Get a second opinion.
- At a minimum, basic tests for unusual 'chabdominal' discomfort should be ordered including an electrocardiogram, chest x-ray, and blood tests – even in those who have few or no known risk factors for heart disease.

- Women are at equal risk to men for heart disease, though they tend to develop heart disease at an older age than men.
- As many as one-third of heart attack sufferers report not having any chest pain at all. Those who lack chest discomfort tend to seek help later, are more likely to be older, are treated less aggressively, are at greater risk for misdiagnosis, and are more likely to die in the short-term compared with folks who report the presence of chest pain.
- Women, the elderly and diabetics are prone to have a heart attack without reporting the symptom of chest discomfort.
- Unrecognized heart attack in the elderly is more prevalent based upon cardiac MRI studies in diabetics and non diabetics over age 75.
- The first electrocardiogram is frequently normal or non-diagnostic in heart attack sufferers. Special blood tests also can be within normal limits in the earliest stages of a heart attack. That is why a minimum of eight to 12 hours of observation and repeat testing and monitoring is ideal despite increasing pressure on emergency room doctors to get patients out of the ER quickly as possible.
- Carry in your wallet or purse a laminated, miniature copy of a baseline EKG. It can prove to be priceless. Doctors can compare a new tracing to the old one, searching for changes.
- Know your vital numbers. Record your resting heart rate and blood pressure every year on your birthday, if not monthly.

Ignorance is Not Bliss

Forget the Hollywood version of a heart attack. You know the script – a fat, bald, old man suddenly clutches his chest in agony then collapses to the ground. Don't forget the part where a passerby puffs into his mouth and presses his chest twice. The victim then sits up, coughs a few times and says, "I'm hungry, let's go eat." On a serious note, heart disease causes over 250,000 sudden deaths annually in the United States and can be quite dramatic. Many of the 900,000 or so heart attacks each year in the United States (and many more worldwide) are less dramatic and far more subtle.

Are you at higher risk for a heart attack? Some myths to dispel: A heart attack victim does not have to be overweight, does not have to be old, does not have to be male, and does not have to have crushing chest pain. In fact, there may be few, if any, chest symptoms in up to one-third of heart attacks, as mentioned earlier. Many more people will seek care at hospital emergency rooms with chest discomfort that proves to be early or stable heart disease or some ailment unrelated to the heart.

The first step in this process is to be aware of any risk factors you might have for heart attack.

Risk Factors One Cannot Change (check all those that apply to you)

□ Older age: As more years pass by, heart disease risk increases

□ Men have greater risk for heart disease at a younger age; risk for women goes way up after menopause

□ Family history of heart disease

□ Race (African Americans, American Indians, and Mexican Americans are more likely to develop heart disease than Caucasians

Risk Factors that can be Changed and Improved (check all those that apply to you)

Studies have estimated that heart attack risk can be reduced by as much as *80 percent* through aggressive risk factor modification:

□ Smoking more than doubles the risk for heart attack.

□ High levels of bad cholesterol (LDL) and low levels of good cholesterol (HDL) may increase risk.

□ High blood pressure that remains uncontrolled even with diet, exercise and drug treatment.

□ The couch potato with low levels of physical activity is playing a dangerous game heart-wise.

□ Obesity, defined as more than 20 percent above one's ideal body weight, ups the heart disease ante. A more accurate risk measure is waist circumference above 40 inches (102 cm) in men and above 35 inches (89 cm) in women. Waist circumference measurement is one feature of the undesirable metabolic syndrome which includes high triglyceride levels, low good cholesterol (HDL) levels, the body's inability to use insulin efficiently, and an elevated blood pressure.

□ Diabetes is a major risk factor for cardiovascular disease. Uncontrolled diabetes poses serious risk for heart damage.

□ High levels of C-reactive protein (CRP) in the blood is a rough measure of active inflammation in the body and may up risk for cardiac events.

□ Extreme stress and anger can provoke sudden heart damage (Broken Heart Syndrome)

□ Cocaine or amphetamine abuse can trigger a heart attack even in young folks.

Lesser Known Risk Factors for Heart Disease (check all those that apply to you)

□ **Left Ventricular Hypertrophy (LVH):** Thickening of the left ventricle, the heart's major blood-pumping chamber, has been identified as a risk factor for heart attack, stroke and death. Heart muscle thickening usually results from high blood pressure or blocked arteries and can be diagnosed accurately on an echocardiogram (sonogram of the heart). Treatments are available once identified.

□ **Heart Rate**: Resting heart rate above 80-85 beats per minute can boost risk for heart disease and death from all causes.

□ **Kidney Disease**: Chronic kidney disease with aging has been strongly linked to ticker trouble.

□ **Atrial Fibrillation**: This erratic, irregular beating of the smaller heart chambers now affects over 35 million people worldwide. With the aging world population, one in four people will suffer from atrial fibrillation at some point in life. Those who have this irregular heart rhythm have 5 times the risk of suffering a stroke. Recent studies show greater peril for heart attacks as well.

□ **Pneumonia:** Hospital admissions for pneumonia are associated with more heart arrhythmias and worse heart outcomes both during and *after* hospitalization, according to one recent study.

□ **Orthostatic Hypotension**: A significant drop in blood pressure when standing up is a common concern in the elderly. When blood pressure goes too low it can cause dizziness, weakness, fainting and falls. Several studies confirm that a drop in standing blood pressure ups chances for stroke, heart attack and death from all causes. What causes this drop in blood pressure on standing? Hospitalization, dehydration, prolonged bed rest, blood pressure medications and diseases such as Parkinson's or diabetes can predispose people to this dangerous drop in blood pressure.

□ **Periodontal Disease:** Diseases of the gums (poor oral hygiene) leads to increased body inflammation which triggers greater propensity for clots to form in heart arteries. This can raise heart disease risk.

□ **High Sugar Diet**: A recent study based upon data from the National Health and Nutrition Examination Survey covering a study period from 1988 to 2010 found that adults whose dietary sugar intake exceeds 25 percent of total calories have a threefold higher risk for heart disease.

The "Hollywood" and "Textbook" Heart Attack

In drama shows, a heart attack is depicted as a middle-aged, overweight man suddenly clutching his chest, getting flustered then collapsing to the ground – dead. Most heart attacks are nothing like this. Each person must understand the textbook signs and symptoms of serious angina or a heart attack. The first major clue is sudden chest, back or abdominal area (Chabdominal) *discomfort* that comes on bad and soon changes to worse with increasing intensity over several minutes. Each person perceives and describes that 'discomfort' differently. Several other symptoms often accompany that primary discomfort including any combination of breathing difficulty, soaking sweats, heart pounding or racing, nausea or vomiting, diarrhea, severe fatigue, unusual anxiety or sense of impending doom, dizziness or fainting. That mid-torso discomfort can also send signals of displeasure to the shoulders, arms, neck, jaw or back.

The "Less Typical" Heart Attack is More Typical

Many heart attacks are far less obvious and dramatic than the textbook or Hollywood variety of ticker damage. Older folks, diabetics and women are more likely to have less typical symptoms of a heart attack like absence of so-called chest pain. Other vague 'chabdominal' (chest or abdominal) complaints may occur but are not described as chest pain. Other frequent major complaints in those with active heart trouble are:

- Breathing trouble
- Extreme fatigue or weakness
- Nausea and vomiting
- Soaking sweats
- Unfamiliar mid to upper backache
- Unfamiliar indigestion
- Unusual severe anxiety and unwell feeling, often perceived as dread or impending doom. Caution: ER doctors often dismiss this as "nerves" or panic attack and send these folks home.
- Loss of functional ability in frail old folks such as new confusion or sudden inability to walk or get out of bed.
- Sudden loss of appetite or loss of function in the elderly

Features that Make Heart Trouble or Heart Attack *More* Likely

The following features of illness should prop your eyes open wide and inch your index finger closer to numbers 9-1-1 on your phone:

- Chest or abdominal area (Chabdominal) discomfort— if there is any at all— that is unlike anything you have ever felt. It comes on strong and grows stronger over a few minutes. Any exertion such as walking can bring on or intensify heart-related discomfort.
- A group of symptoms that occur in short order and in any combination along with chabdominal discomfort. To reiterate, these secondary symptoms might include breathing trouble, racing heart, drenching sweats, nausea or vomiting, diarrhea, dizziness or fainting, extreme weakness, or unusual anxiety.
- Having a history of heart disease, diabetes, high blood pressure, kidney disease, or other chronic illnesses. Presence of risk factors for heart disease should set a lower threshold for seeking immediate emergency medical care.

- Older age. Let's face it, the older you are chances go way up unusual discomfort is ominous.
- Abnormal vital signs such as high or low blood pressure or pulse rate or rapid breathing during an episode of "chabdominal" discomfort should raise red flags.

Features that Make Heart Trouble or Heart Attack *Less* Likely

- 'Chabdominal' (chin, chest or abdominal area) discomfort that starts up or gets worse with a deep breath in or while coughing.
- Chabdominal discomfort that starts up or gets worse with twisting your torso and arms from side to side, suggesting a muscle or rib injury. Tenderness when pressing on an area of the rib cage should not itself exclude a heart condition. Press hard enough and anybody would feel pain with this maneuver that doctors use to check for costochondritis, an inflammation in the ribcage area.
- The symptoms you feel now are *identical* to those when you were given a *definitive* diagnosis in the past such as gallbladder attack, kidney stone, lung infection or muscle pull, to name a few. Definitive here means significant testing was done with clearly positive results confirming that past diagnosis.
- Fleeting chest area discomfort that lasts under five seconds then resolves is less likely a heart problem. Same with chest area discomfort that stays with you *constantly* for days.

Heart Disease: Special Considerations in the Elderly

Older and frail folks can easily fool loved ones and doctors with their many ailments. Heart problems are no exception. Older people might have a higher pain threshold, can have limitations in communicating illness, might be reluctant to bother a caregiver, or may resist telling someone about illness out of fear of dying at the hospital or being sent to a nursing home. What's more, older folks have other diseases that could be used to explain away vague symptoms during a heart attack. Signs of a heart attack in frail folks can be subtle and include:

- Confusion
- Sudden loss of functional ability
- Apathy
- Vague feeling of unwellness
- Self-neglect
- Vomiting or loss of appetite
- Unexplained fall
- Breathing trouble or suddenly worsening heart failure
- Increased fatigue or weakness

Silent or Unrecognized Heart Attacks: Shockingly More Common than Previously Thought

A recent study used MRI testing of the heart in a population of older adults in Iceland. What they discovered is a bit frightening. Researchers identified more heart damage evidence for silent or unrecognized heart attacks than damage from known, symptomatic and diagnosed attacks. "Silent" heart attack is well-described in diabetics who have nerve damage that blunts symptoms. But some experts theorize a temporary blockage of a heart-feeding artery may cause mild heart scarring but blood flow is naturally reestablished quickly enough. The sufferer would then experience few, if any, symptoms. This process, it is believed, might serve as a middle step on the path to full-blown heart attack crises. Another key factor in unrecognized ticker trouble is the less typical symptom complex that fools both patients and doctors into misdiagnosis of an actual mild attack (see above). This is ever more common in older folks. In fact, the majority of all heart attacks were either silent or unrecognized, according to this and other studies. There was a higher death risk even for silent heart disease. This underscores the need for people to learn the *subtle presentations* of this common killer and identify when adults need to see a doctor for masked heart disease.

If properly identified, these folks can get appropriate early treatment to prevent future catastrophic events. More concerning is the estimate that as many as 80 percent of episodes of insufficient nourishment to the heart (ischemia) show no symptoms at all. Absent is the expected angina discomfort, breathing trouble, arm pain. One previous study found that as many as 10 to 40 percent of older folks with no prior history of heart disease showed evidence of silent starvation of needed nutrients to the heart, known as *ischemia*. Ischemia is the stepping stone to a full-blown heart attack or sudden death. Those who had uncontrolled high blood pressure or leg artery disease were more likely to experience silent heart ischemia (nutrient starvation). Unfortunately, searching for classic symptoms of a heart problem and performing a simple electrocardiogram are often insufficient to make an accurate diagnosis.

Missed Opportunity: Early Warning Symptoms Often Ignored

Doctors always say that patients must learn the signs and symptoms of heart attack. They also stress the importance of carefully discerning whether someone with chest area discomfort truly has heart disease or some other ailment like gastritis or ulcer. Practically speaking, once a person is 40 years of age or older, it is prudent to dispel the myth that speaking to a patient and doing a quick physical examination can "rule out" a heart-related cause for chest discomfort. Forget about it! Recall that heart attack sufferers often describe chest area symptoms as 'heartburn' and as many as one-third of those afflicted with heart disease deny having chest area discomfort at all! To reiterate, this is particularly true for older folks, women and diabetics. Splitting hairs on a diagnosis is difficult when sick people give vague descriptions and older folks with communication difficulty cannot say much at all about their illness. The simple **solution:** Take any persistent, severe or unusual symptom or ailment seriously if over age 40. It should be considered possible heart disease until proven otherwise. Why is heart disease the default diagnosis? Cardiovascular illness can be tricky, subtle and easily missed; moreover, it remains the number one killer across the globe. Heart disease can kill in the blink of an eye.

Instead of splitting hairs about a diagnosis, people should look for great big neon signs! Little is ever spoken about the earliest warning signs heart attack sufferers commonly experience in the days to months *prior* to a full-blown attack. These early symptoms are perhaps analogous to the TIA that we now know serves as code-red warning sign for an imminent, catastrophic stroke (see also, Stroke Chapter).

Many studies have shown that heart attack sufferers, when asked, reported feeling unusual symptoms for days to weeks to months *prior* to the main event. These ill feelings were either brand new or noticeably worse than they had ever experienced prior. Sadly, the vague nature of these sensations leads people to ignore them. With no chest pain, there is no heart attack, right? Wrong answer. When those suffering warning signs of heart disease seek medical care, doctors often downplay their symptoms and miss an early diagnosis opportunity. These symptoms frequently recur daily in the days to weeks before the full-blown event. Take note: The most commonly reported *advance warning* symptoms experienced by heart attack sufferers *before* the main attack are as follows:

- Extreme or unusual **fatigue** that is more persistent than having a bad day or two. This weakness, of course, cannot be easily explained by common problems like an obvious viral infection or known anemia, for instance.
- Nagging and unfamiliar **pain or discomfort** in the chest or abdominal area ('chabdominal'), mid-back under the shoulder blades, neck, arms and shoulders, jaw or throat. Do not assume, without a fall or exercise injury, that these persistent aches and pains are just a muscle strain or arthritis. Don't let your doctor reflexively dismiss the problem as minor, despite that being the answer you would want to hear.
- Severe or unusual **anxiety** can be another early warning sign of imminent heart attack, unless you are about to get married, start a difficult job, or experience some other clearly stressful event. Without a logical precipitant or history of similar mental health issues, get a heart evaluation if stricken by unusual anxiety or a feeling of impending doom. On the other hand, severe anger or mental anguish can cause heart damage – the Broken Heart Syndrome. Interestingly, women often report significant **sleep difficulties** for days to weeks prior to suffering a heart attack. If persistent insomnia is unusual for you, it may be prudent to see your doctor for a

heart evaluation! Do not just accept a sleeping pill prescription as you get rushed out the door.

- **Stomach-related** problems are commonly experienced prior to a major coronary event. They can include unusual feelings of heartburn or indigestion or episodes of nausea and vomiting. Sudden, unexplained **loss of appetite** can also manifest prior to "the big one."
- **Head-related** ailments can include dizziness, unusual headache and vision disturbances.
- Episodes of unexplained **shortness of breath** or racing heart can also appear days to weeks prior to a major attack.

To reiterate, these vague, advance-warning symptoms tend to recur *daily* for days to weeks before a major coronary event! If your unusual symptoms do not resolve in a couple of days, it is prudent to get evaluated for heart disease by your family doctor or a cardiologist. The evaluation should include taking a history, an examination, vital signs, and testing such as EKG, blood tests, chest x-ray. More elaborate heart tests like stress test, echocardiogram and others might prove necessary if symptoms persist or if a basic test shows even minor abnormalities. The neon signs of an impending heart attack might be in plain view, waiting for you to read them and take action.

Because these red flag symptoms can be vague, each person must learn to *listen* to his or her own body. Perhaps silent heart attack is actually a culmination of several factors including patient denial, atypical symptoms, misdiagnosis by doctor, difficult to interpret EKG, reduced pain perception in the elderly and diabetics, as well as incorrect labeling of the cause for symptoms as indigestion, being over-tired or similar excuses. This theory has not been proven.

Invasive Treatments for Heart Attack

Riskier heart attack treatments like clot-dissolving drugs or balloon-opening of clogged arteries followed by stent implantation do have clear and proven benefits. Unfortunately, these time-dependent, invasive treatments can lead to catastrophic complications in the elderly. Older folks are more susceptible to serious complications because of a delicate health balance called frailty, their many chronic illnesses, taking multiple medications and reduced kidney function. As time passes from onset of heart attack symptoms until definitive invasive treatment, the benefit of these treatments plummets. It is estimated that three million stents are implanted worldwide into people's heart arteries each year. Just a few key points about these invasive and risky treatments:

- Treatment with balloon device (PCI) opening of the clotted artery and placement of a stent (a metal bridge to prop open arteries) must be initiated within 90 minutes of symptom onset for maximal benefit; Clot-dissolving medication can still be effective if given within 12 hours of symptom onset.
- Less than one-third of United States hospitals offer balloon device opening treatment (PCI), a therapy uniformly considered *most* effective for heart attack. Find out which hospitals in your area offer this treatment and how successful their ranking is by checking state Health Department websites.
- Balloon device opening of arteries is commonly overused in folks who suffer from less severe heart disease without an active heart attack. This has been labeled the 'oculostenotic reflex,' meaning cardiologists see a fixed plaque narrowing in a heart-feeding artery and reflexively want to open that narrowing. Patients also logically want to unclog the arterial pipe as they would a blocked sink drain. That is not, however, how heart attacks work! A plumber opens a clogged pipe and all is well again; arteries are more complicated than simple pipes. A 20 percent plaque-blocked artery can lead to heart attack before a 60 percent blocked artery. It is now well established that people who have predictable angina symptoms (stable heart disease) do *no better* with regard to heart attack and death risk whether treated with balloon-device opening of a blockage (PCI) or just effective drug treatment, proper diet and moderate exercise.
- Drs. Nallamothu and Krumholz have recently raised the concern that cardiologists routinely do balloon-opening and stent procedures right after the angiogram is done to get an initial diagnosis. This one-two punch of diagnosis then treatment is clearly appropriate

for heart emergencies, but might lead to overuse of stents in people with stable heart symptoms. If the stent procedure is routinely *delayed* for a future day, the doctors argue in a 2010 *Journal of the American Medical Association* commentary, both doctor and patient can more leisurely discuss angiogram findings for stable heart disease. Less risky treatment options such as medication, exercise and proper diet can be given an opportunity to work before the heavy treatment guns are used.

- It is concerning that proper informed consent for stent procedures may be lacking. A 2010 study surveyed 153 people. These participants consented to an elective angiogram to evaluate the heart arteries and to undergo possible balloon opening and stent procedures as well. The majority of these people, it turns out, *incorrectly* believed the procedure would *lower risk for death and heart attack* even though they had stable heart disease. What is more concerning, a 2014 study published in the *Journal of the American Medical Association Internal Medicine* surveyed cardiologists on their discussions with patients about angiograms and stents for stable heart disease. Ninety-five percent of the heart specialists did *not* tell the patients that stent procedures do *not* lower chances for death or heart attack when performed outside of a heart attack emergency situation! Some doctors in this survey incorrectly told stable patients that a stent would actually *prevent* a future heart attack. Other doctors admitted they did procedures to allay fear in patients because people believe unclogging a pipe leads to better results. This is not the case with complex heart arteries and risky procedures that open up these clogged arteries.
- Pretty amazing that many people are misled into undergoing risky procedures for non-emergency heart disease because some doctors exaggerate benefits of the procedure or use technical jargon that patients misunderstand. If patients only knew that studies have confirmed that proper diet and exercise *does better* than getting risky PCI procedures. Dr Rainer Hambrecht and colleagues did an analysis of over 200 stable heart patients randomly assigned to receive either the invasive stent procedure or a moderate intensity exercise program. Patients in the exercise program did better than

those getting a procedure. This result makes sense since opening a blockage in an artery with a stent temporarily solves a problem in one small section; exercising and proper dieting reduces body inflammation and other negative factors to tip the balance away from heart attack-causing clots in the *entire* arterial system.

- Beware of invasive heart procedures outside of an emergency situation. A 2011 review of 145,000 elective heart procedures from the National Cardiovascular Data Registry found about half the elective procedures to be *inappropriate*! It is always wise to get a second opinion before undergoing a risky elective procedure. In truth, it is not uncommon for cardiologists to overstate the benefits of implanting a heart stent for stable patients.
- Problems with inappropriate heart procedures are not limited to elective procedures in stable patients. One recent report found that over one-third of patients referred from the emergency department for a stent procedure did not, in fact, have a major heart attack most amenable to stent treatment. Contributing factors for this inappropriate referral include the difficulty in diagnosing heart attack in people who do not complain of chest pain, and preexisting electrocardiogram abnormalities that further cloud the diagnosis of heart attack.
- Serious risks posed by clot-busting medication or stent implantation procedures include life-threatening bleeding, kidney failure, heart attack, serious irregular heartbeat, stroke and death.
- Severe headache can be the sole complaint experienced by some elderly heart attack sufferers.
- With three million stents being implanted worldwide each year, the risk of stent thrombosis is becoming a problem of public health proportions, according to a cardiology journal.

A Few Heart Disease Pearls

- Studies published in the *New England Journal of Medicine* and other journals have found a heart attack diagnosis is missed in about 2 of 100 heart attack patients seeking help in United States emergency rooms, in 3 of 100 heart attack patients in Canada, and in 6 of 100 heart attack sufferers in United Kingdom emergency rooms.

- Patients who suffer a heart attack without experiencing chest area discomfort are more likely to delay seeking care, more often are misdiagnosed and have twice the risk of death while in the hospital than those who do describe chest pains as a heart attack symptom.
- There is some evidence that people create mental templates of common diseases based upon knowledge of common symptoms associated with those diseases. That knowledge may come from public education campaigns, Hollywood depictions or life experiences. When acutely ill, people compare their own symptoms to those disease templates to self-diagnose. This is why this info is crucial. Public education campaigns tend to over-simplify signs and symptoms; Hollywood depictions of illness are usually way off base. The result: inaction when less typical signs and symptoms of heart disease are ignored or dismissed.
- According to Dr. John Morley, Chairman of Geriatrics at Saint Louis University, the elderly are less likely to complain of chest pain with acute heart disease and more likely to describe feeling winded with walking or other exertion. Burning sensations in the upper abdomen or chest area might be described as well.
- Dr. Jean McSweeney, PhD Program Director at the University of Arkansas, studied **early warning symptoms** in *women* who suffered a heart attack. The most common symptoms that these women experienced for days to weeks before the major event include insomnia; unusual anxiety; severe fatigue; stomach complaints (nausea, indigestion, loss of appetite); headache, vision disturbances or dizziness; sweating or racing heart; breathing difficulty; and pains in areas as diverse as chest, shoulders or shoulder blade area, arm, neck, jaw, legs. Study participants said they experienced their early-warning symptoms almost every day for a period of time just before the heart attack.
- These early warning symptoms before a heart attack may not have been emphasized, according to some sources, because of fear emergency departments might get inundated with false alarms. After

all, many of these symptoms like fatigue and insomnia might affect everybody at some point. However, that is why chest pain units have been set up in hospitals. These units are prepared to separate out high-risk from low-risk patients who are concerned about heart disease. Those with risk factors such as smoking, diabetes, hypertension and strong family history for heart disease should be most alert to persistent early-warning signs of heart disease.

- It is not uncommon for a heart attack sufferer to experience some precipitant like mental anguish or severe anger or strenuous exercise prior to a heart attack. Of note, heart attacks occur frequently between 6 AM and 12 noon.
- For those who do experience chest pain, general guidelines suggest usual *stable angina* pain lasts about 2 to 10 minutes; unstable angina typically lasts 10 to 30 minutes and heart attack chest pain lasts longer than 30 minutes.
- Reminder: Any chabdominal discomfort (from chin to chest to lower abdomen, or back) that is unusual or severe enough to make you stop your routine needs to be taken seriously. Do not deny, just comply. Seek help… or maybe say goodbye.
- Anxiety should never be an acceptable diagnosis given in an emergency room setting. Serious diagnoses like heart disease, lung disease, or abdominal cavity ailments must be excluded first before even considering anxiety as final diagnosis.
- When testing is performed in an emergency room, specifically ask your doctor if results are totally normal or uncertain and non-diagnostic. There is a huge difference between the two as to how closely you must follow up on your illness.
- Delays in seeking care for sudden illness are commonly rooted in fear of being seriously ill and denial that symptoms suggest heart attack or stroke or abdominal crisis. It is easier to maintain this self-deception charade in isolation by taking a nap and praying it will all be gone when you awaken. My advice: first speak with a trusted friend or relative and describe the problem. Most likely, your symptoms will appear to be far more sinister from their vantage point and they will try to snap you out from your stupor

of denial and fear. Do NOT go to sleep when feeling severe and unusual symptoms.

- Following is a checklist of questions to ask yourself when unusual and severe illness stops your routine. If you answer "yes" to any of these then seek help asap:
    * Am I over age 40?
    * Any risks for heart disease?
    * Are my current symptoms, taken together, some of the worst feelings I have ever experienced?
    * Any chabdominal discomfort symptoms (chin to chest, abdomen, back)?
    * Am I experiencing *grouped symptoms*, meaning several symptoms all at once like breathing trouble, nausea or vomiting, profuse sweats, racing heart, feeling of impending doom, dizziness or faint feeling?
    * Is pain traveling around into back, shoulders, arms, abdomen?
    * If you are worried about calling for an ambulance or making a fuss, at least tell a friend and ask for a ride to the emergency room.
    * If you must maintain control of your situation, avoid labeling your problem with false diagnoses like "It's just heartburn." If you truly are the take-charge controlling personality type, then take control of your life and well-being by getting emergency care immediately!

Bear in mind that during a crisis, our mind gets foggy, reasoning may become impaired, vision might get narrow or blurred, and we may feel numb and fatigued. The tendency is to act automatically without clear thinking. Only one thing might save us: ask for help. Tell someone you are feeling ill. Get a friendly opinion. Your decision to deny, minimize and ignore might be your last.

III. DON'T STROKE OUT: UNDERSTANDING, PREVENTING AND IDENTIFYING STROKE — A NOVEL APPROACH

> *When Gregor Samsa woke up one morning from unsettling dreams, he found himself changed in his bed into a monstrous vermin... His many legs... were waving helplessly before his eyes. "What happened to me?" he thought. It was no dream... No matter how hard he threw himself onto his right side, he always rocked onto his back again...*
>
> *"Why don't I keep sleeping for a little while longer and forget all this foolishness?" he thought...*
>
> *...Gregor was startled when he heard his voice answering. It was clearly and unmistakably his earlier voice, but in it was intermingled... painful squeaking which left the words positively distinct only in the first moment and distorted them in the reverberation, so that one didn't know if one had heard correctly.*

In his classic novella, *The Metamorphosis*, Franz Kafka meant to reflect the absurdity and alienation of life. The opening scene, however, might well depict a person awakening with a stroke in progress: limitations with movement and strange body alienation; speech changes and difficulty speaking or understanding; denial that something is amiss; a major metamorphosis of body and brain caused by a sudden, unpredictable event; and a predilection for stroke to occur during the early waking hours.

Consider the following insightful description of a stroke:

> *And then, again, my left hemisphere comes online and it says, "Hey! You've got to pay attention. We've got to get help." And I'm thinking, "I got to get help. I gotta focus." So I get out of the shower and I mechanically dress and I'm walking around my apartment, and I'm thinking, "I gotta get to work. I gotta get to work. Can I drive? Can I drive?"*

> *...And in that moment my right arm went totally paralyzed by my side. Then I realized, "Oh my gosh! I'm having a stroke! I'm having a stroke!"*
>
> *...Eventually, the whole number gets dialed and I'm listening to the phone, and my colleague picks up the phone and he says to me, "Woo woo woo woo." And I think to myself, "Oh my gosh, he sounds like a Golden Retriever!"*
>
> *And so I say to him — clear in my mind, I say to him: "This is Jill! I need help!" And what comes out of my voice is, "Woo woo woo woo woo." I'm thinking, "Oh my gosh, I sound like a Golden Retriever." So I couldn't know — I didn't know that I couldn't speak or understand language until I tried. So he recognizes that I need help and he gets me help.*

These riveting excerpts from neuroscientist Jill Bolte-Taylor's description of her stroke experience at age 37 offer insight into the left-brain havoc and body devastation of a stroke. I urge you to read her stroke description in its entirety or to hear her talk on Ted.com using this link: http://www.ted.com/talks/jill_bolte_taylor_s_powerful_stroke_of_insight?language=en

Unlike Ms. Taylor's experience, strokes that devastate the *right* side of the brain can cause left arm and leg paralysis and a bizarre syndrome of total neglect of the left side of the body and left visual field perception. Jenni Ogden, PhD, a clinical neuropsychologist, wrote the following description of hemineglect in *Psychology Today.*

> *...the patient sat in her wheelchair with her head screwed around as far to the right as possible, and refused to look or speak to me if I stood on her left side. She would eat only the food off the right side of her plate, and she refused to acknowledge that her left arm and leg belonged to her.*

As these cases illustrate, nobody would want to spend the rest of his or her life afflicted with a debilitating stroke syndrome. The most devastating consequences of stroke are paralysis of an entire side of the body; loss of ability to speak or understand language (aphasia), making communication with others difficult and frustrating; loss of ability to write and read; loss of memory (dementia); and loss of bladder and bowel control.

Following are several bizarre and less common consequences of suffering specific types of strokes:

- Alien Hand Syndrome – Sufferers report that an affected hand has a mind of its own and performs tasks out of their control.
- Foreign Accent Syndrome – Sufferers suddenly speak with a foreign accent.
- Brain Blindness – Brain attack victims lose sight from damage to vision wiring in the brain, yet they deny they cannot see.
- Hemi-neglect – Wherein a brain attack affecting the right brain causes paralysis of the left arm and leg and sufferers deny that the stricken arm and leg belong to them!
- Prosopognosia – Loss of ability to recognize faces and emotional expressions including not recognizing family and friends by appearance.
- Apraxia – Loss of ability to perform purposeful tasks. For instance, putting on shoes before socks or trying to write with a knife.
- Tactile Agnosia – Loss of ability to recognize familiar objects by touch.

Unlike the many helpful treatments available for heart attacks, aspirin and blood pressure control are the only proven safe and effective treatments for most strokes. Clot-dissolving treatment has gained momentum in the treatment of evolving strokes but remains quite controversial regarding the balance scale of high-stakes risks versus possible benefit.

Warning! Pay close attention to what follows or you might one day be hitching a ride in an ambulance to a nearby emergency room – like Gregor Samsa in *The Metamorphosis* – changed forever.

What is a stroke?

If one considers arteries as copper pipes, strokes are caused by two types of plumbing problems: clogged arteries and leaky arteries. About 80 percent of strokes are caused by a clog in an artery that feeds oxygen and nutrients to any part of the brain (ischemic). Brain cells in that area begin to die when the blood spigot is shut off – a stroke in progress – and depending on the function of those brain cells, different symptoms and signs develop. An artery springing a leak (hemorrhagic) is responsible for about 15 percent of strokes as blood floods the brain and injures nearby brain cells.

As a general rule, clogging of an artery in the *heart* causes a heart attack; artery blockage in the *brain* causes a stroke. But what is important to understand is that heart attacks are primarily one type of disease. Hardening of arteries and inflammation can lead to a blood clot shutting off blood flow in a heart-feeding artery. Stroke, however, is several different diseases lumped under one name. Hardening of arteries can occur in brain arteries, leading to a blockage and stroke. A clot forms in the diseased brain artery and eventually shuts off blood flow like a clogged drain. But a traveling clot (embolism) can form in the neck and other arteries, or even the heart itself. This clot breaks away and travels to a brain artery, suddenly cutting off blood flow in the brain like corking a wine bottle while wine is flowing into a glass. Different plugged up brain arteries will cause very different symptoms and function losses.

Hemorrhagic strokes (blood leaking into the brain) have completely different causes such as an aneurysm or skyrocketing blood pressure. Stroke is surely a group of different diseases which might explain why many treatments that work well for heart attacks do *not* necessarily work so well for strokes (see also, clot-dissolving drugs, below).

Some Sobering Statistics

Strokes can have devastating consequences for the sufferer, burdened family members, and the healthcare system. Most patients who survive a heart attack will walk out of the hospital – after the obligatory wheelchair ride to the front door – and try to resume a normal life by improving lifestyle and perhaps taking many medications. Not so with stroke sufferers who survive. Many survivors are bed- or chair-bound for life. They need assistance with daily life activities such as dressing or toileting or preparing food. They develop depression and frustration due to limited mobility or loss of limb function. They may experience permanent communication difficulties affecting speech, language, writing, reading and vision. Brain attack victims also suffer from complications such as pneumonia, bedsores, pain, muscle spasm, swallowing challenges that make eating favorite foods difficult, loss of quality of life, memory loss and many other devastating consequences.

The statistics:

- By far the most important stat: **Up to 80 percent of strokes are preventable**, according to the National Stroke Association!
- The World Health Organization estimates there are 15 million strokes worldwide every year. About 5 million strokes result in permanent disability.
- Each year, nearly 800,000 Americans suffer a stroke; 50,000 Australians have the same fate; 150,000 people in the United Kingdom are stroke-stricken; and about 50,000 Canadians suffer a "brain attack."
- Approximately 20 to 30 percent of strokes prove to be fatal.
- It has been estimated that for each hour of evolving stroke, the injured brain loses about 3.6 years worth of brain cells that would have died with normal aging.
- Between one-half and two-thirds of stroke victims have disability that impedes some activities of daily living, rendering those people forever dependent on others for help.
- Boomers beware! Approximately one-fourth of strokes strike people *under* age 65.
- There are about 650,000 stroke deaths every year in Europe, according to the World Health Report 2002 (WHO).
- Stroke is a leading cause of long-term, permanent disability worldwide.
- Brain attack sufferers are at nine-fold greater risk for developing **dementia**. In fact, about one in four stroke victims develop signs of memory loss within one year.

- You may have to read this stat twice to believe it: New research gleaned from high quality MRI and CT scan testing in recent years has found that devastating strokes discussed above are merely the tip of the iceberg! Ninety-five percent of strokes actually go *unnoticed* – the silent stroke! More about these subtle but devastating strokes on the website at **www.emergencyroomsurvivalbookforolderadults.com**.

"Don't Stroke Out" – A New Stroke Education Approach

This **Don't Stroke Out** program strives to inform people around the globe about stroke dangers using terms and concepts that are familiar to many people. People can recall images more easily than piles of facts. A concept-based or image-based approach can surely help improve memory of major stroke risks, signs and symptoms.

This program also emphasizes helping people to understand the devastating effects of stroke through riveting anecdotes, actual video and media accounts, and references from the arts and literature. Stroke is not just an amorphous disease that strikes old, decrepit people; it is a life-changer that robs people of their quality of life, independence, productivity, ability to speak, communicate, read, write, see and remember.

For many stroke victims, hugging loved ones or uttering the words "I love you" may never again be possible.

Stroke commonly causes a return to the dependence of infancy, akin to *The Curious Case of Benjamin Button*, a short story written by F. Scott Fitzgerald in 1922 in which a man ages backwards from old age to infancy. Many stroke sufferers must eventually be fed, have diapers changed, and get moved from bed to chair to wheelchair by a caregiver. And that is if the stroke sufferer even survives!

"Stroke" to many folks remains a vague concept that affects only hunched, frail grandmas and grandpas and does not really apply to them. Recall the statistic above that up to 25 percent of strokes occur in those *under* age 65! Sadly, recent surveys confirm that most people have trouble naming more than one key feature of a stroke. How, then, will they be able to identify a brain attack in progress and seek help? What's more, without knowing risk factors, how will these folks live a lifestyle everyday that minimizes chances they wind up on a permanent wheelchair ride dressed in diapers?

Strike One: Stroke Risk Factors

Every individual has a different genetic makeup and lifestyle that either increases stroke risk or is protective. Some risk factors for stroke such as older age cannot be changed; Genetic makeup was once in the unchangeable category, but recent research suggests that proper diet can have gene-modifying effects and thus reduce heart attack and possibly stroke risk. About 25 percent of the population carries two copies of a gene variant called 9p21. Studies have shown these people have a significantly increased risk for heart attacks (and possibly strokes), but this high-risk gene can perhaps be "turned off" by eating a healthful diet.

What is clear is that everyone over age 40 should make a careful assessment of their medical conditions, diet and lifestyle to evaluate their stroke risk. Recall that up to 80 percent of strokes are preventable, according to the National Stroke Association. So don't stroke out!

Stroke Risk Factors that *Cannot* be Changed

You cannot change your sex, age, family history or ethnicity; however, your brow should be raised, eyes widened, and ears perked up if you fit into some of these risk categories. It is you who must work hardest on the risk factors you *can* control to minimize your stroke risk.

- Increasing **Age**
- **Men** generally have a greater stroke risk than women
- **Family history** of stroke poses some undefined greater brain attack risk
- **Race**: African Americans and Hispanics are at greater risk for stroke and death from stroke
- **Genes**: A documented stroke in a parent before age 65 triples brain attack risk in children, the Framingham Study has shown.

- **Memory Loss** has been found to pose a twofold increased risk for stroke in the elderly

Stroke Risk Factors that *Can* be Changed

These are the risk factors that are in *your* hands. You can slash your risk for a brain attack by changing habits and lifestyle. Ignore this at your own peril. You can minimize your chances for a life of wheelchairs, bedpans and frustration. Stroke may not happen next week if you continue a high-risk lifestyle. Perhaps it is years away. But today is the best day to optimize a stroke-free lifestyle. Learn the risks. Learn the signs. But don't stroke out!

The Risk Factors You Can Control (check risks that apply to you)

- □ **Cigarette Smoking** – A no-brainer risk that can and should be eliminated. Second-hand smoke might also increase risk of a brain attack. Smoking, in fact, has been identified in studies as a leading risk factor for the dreaded and severe hemorrhagic (leaky artery) stroke.
- □ **High Blood Pressure** (Hypertension) – Possibly the single most important risk factor for stroke, although some strokes are *not* directly related to high blood pressure. Poor diet and being overweight up your chances for having high blood pressure. Blood pressure should be below 140/80-90, but not too low (not under 115/70) in frail elders. It is good practice to measure blood pressure while sitting *and* standing up in older adults.
- □ **Diabetes Mellitus** (High Blood Sugar) – This insidious disease *significantly* increases risk for heart attack, stroke, kidney disease, eye disease, infections and many other serious ailments. Again, poor diet and being overweight magnify chances for having diabetes and are within your control. Very tight blood sugar control, however, is *unlikely* to reduce stroke risk.
- □ **High Blood Cholesterol** – The EPIC Potsdam Study estimated 60 percent of clogged artery (ischemia) stroke risk is attributed to high blood pressure, diabetes, high cholesterol, smoking and excessive alcohol use. Several major studies have found a clear

relationship between higher bad cholesterol level and greater stroke risk. Other studies were less clear on this association. The evidence is generally good for cholesterol, unlike the weaker associations for high triglycerides (type of fat in the blood) and brain attack peril. Clearly, it is preferable to have normal-range blood levels of cholesterol and triglycerides.

- □ **Excessive Alcohol Intake** – The American Heart Association recommends that men indulge in two or fewer drinks daily, while the limit for women is one alcohol indulgence daily.
- □ **Couch Potato Lifestyle** (No exercise) – Moderate exercise offers many benefits including weight reduction, increased muscle mass, decreased stress, lower blood pressure and blood sugar, and reduced body inflammation. Being a sofa-surfer has been shown to up chances for a brain attack by as much as 30 percent. Get up and run for your life! Pick an activity that you enjoy and can maintain – weights, swimming, yard work and gardening, jogging, biking, tennis, tai chi, martial arts – there are many movement activities from which to choose to satisfy all tastes and physical limitations.
- □ **Heart Disease** – Stroke risk is increased in those with heart disease including heart attack, angina, valve abnormalities, enlarged heart, heart failure, heart thickening (Left Ventricular Hypertrophy), and certain birth defects that allow passage of blood between the right and left sides of the heart (Patent Foramen Ovale, Atrial Septal Defect).
- □ **Atrial Fibrillation** – This is a heart disease risk factor that deserves special mention because it *triples* stroke risk. Having many different causes, an uncoordinated contraction of a chamber of the heart (atrium) allows clots to form. This heart rhythm abnormality can affect about one in twenty people over age 70. When atrial-fibrillation-caused clots travel to the brain, they tend to cause larger and more disabling strokes. Blood thinning medications reduce stroke risk, but pros and cons of using blood thinners should be discussed in detail with a doctor.
- □ **Abdominal Obesity** – Fat cells located within abdominal cavity organs (liver, kidneys, intestinal lining, etc) secrete many

chemicals that increase body inflammation and blood thickness, thereby increasing stroke and heart attack risk. One recent study found four times greater stroke risk in men with waistlines above 40 inches and women who had waistlines greater than 35 inches (measured across the belly button).

- □ **Fatty Liver Disease** – A recent study showed a tripling of stroke risk in those who suffer from a little-known disorder called fatty liver disease (fat deposits in the liver). This disorder, part of abdominal obesity, can be diagnosed by abnormal liver enzymes in a standard blood test and by ultrasound. As with abdominal obesity, this disorder contributes to body inflammation and is linked to resistance to the normal actions of the key hormone insulin. Ask your doctor to evaluate you for fatty liver disease.
- □ **Inflammation** – Artery blockages are more than just cholesterol deposits piling up like trash at a dumpsite. Body inflammation is caused by a complex balance of good and bad chemicals produced by fat cells, artery lining (endothelial) cells, and scavenger white blood cells, to name a few. Researchers are finding that many more diseases have root in body inflammation including heart attacks, strokes, asthma and rheumatoid arthritis.
- □ **Significant Infections** – Both acute and chronic infections have been linked to higher risk for a brain attack. Periodontal disease and gingivitis are examples of common chronic infections. Significant chest infections like pneumonia or bronchitis are examples of acute infection. A 2014 report in *Clinical Infectious Diseases* described a significantly elevated risk of stroke in the weeks and months following an attack of Herpes Zoster (shingles). The evidence is unclear, but someone with other risk factors for stroke might consider discussing with their primary care doctor taking a baby aspirin daily for a few weeks after suffering from a serious bout of bronchitis, pneumonia, shingles or flu. Good dental hygiene is of paramount importance as well.
- □ **Obstructive Sleep Apnea** – Partial obstruction of breathing passages during sleep, more common in men and those who are overweight, has been found to be a risk factor for stroke in both

men and women. Risk rises as the severity of the breathing blockage increases.

- □ **Illegal Drugs** – Cocaine and methamphetamine have been shown to up risk of stroke.
- □ **Medications** – Several types of medications can boost risk of stroke or raise blood pressure. Higher risk for stroke: Anti-inflammatory pain relievers such as ibuprofen, naproxen, diclofenac. The Food and Drug Administration has recently emphasized these non-aspirin anti-inflammatory medications as risk factors for heart attack and stroke. Higher doses likely lead to greater risk, especially in those who already have other risk factors; Antipsychotic drugs often overused in the elderly can double risk of death and include risperidone, quetiapine, olanzapine, haloperidol; estrogen-based birth control pills and other hormone supplements. Medications that raise blood pressure include cold remedies containing the decongestant pseudoephedrine. Some cold remedies also have anti-inflammatory ingredients (ibuprofen, naproxen) for pain and fever. Appetite suppressants and special migraine medications can also boost blood pressure levels.
- □ **Diet** – Excessive salt (sodium) intake has been linked to higher blood pressure which can raise stroke risk. Potassium, on the other hand, has been recently found to protect against stroke. A 2014 study of over 90,000 women over age 50, published in the journal *Stroke,* concluded that those who had the highest intake of foods higher in potassium had fewer strokes and lower death rate over the 11-year study period. Foods high in potassium include spinach (175 mg per cup, raw) and other green leafy vegetables, oranges or juice (240 mg), medium-sized banana (425 mg), baked potato (900 mg), sweet potato (450 mg), ¼ cup raisins (270 mg), ½ cup prune juice (350 mg), raw tomato (300 mg), ½ avocado (450 mg). Study participants consumed an average of 2611 mg of potassium daily, falling short of the World Health Organization suggested goal of 3500mg per day. Caution: Those who have significant chronic kidney disease must limit potassium intake based upon their doctor's specific advice.

- □ **Life Stress and Sense of Coherence** – Studies favor an association between stress and stroke risk. The simple proof: There are more strokes and heart attacks in the days after major earthquakes. A recent study that appeared in the *Journal of the American Medical Association* found increased stroke risk after the death of a spouse. Factors such as coping ability, adaptability, ability to make sense of unpredictable life events, and finding meaning can contribute to protection from stroke.
- □ **Living in the "Stroke Belt"** – Eleven states in southeastern United States have been found to have a higher stroke incidence. These states are Alabama, Arkansas, Georgia, Indiana, Kentucky, Louisiana, Mississippi, North Carolina, South Carolina, Tennessee, and Virginia. It is not clear why stroke incidence is higher but theories include a diet higher in fried foods and higher incidence of hypertension in this population.

Strike Two – Stroke Warning!

TIA: Mini-stroke, Maxi-Problem

A transient ischemic attack – popularly known as a TIA or "mini-stroke" – is like angina of the brain. TIA serves as a flashing neon sign to alert the sufferer that there is trouble in paradise. As chest pressure, fatigue and shortness of breath are warning signs of a heart attack waiting to happen, a TIA screams out "beware imminent irreversible brain damage!" Unfortunately, a TIA can be quite subtle, fleeting and difficult even for doctors to diagnose.

Do you tend to ignore your health if a problem comes and goes? Don't want to baby yourself? Well, swing and miss on this pitch and your life will forever be changed. Let's put the past behind us. Forget the smoking and drinking and downing all those cheeseburgers and greasy fries. Ignore the couch potato living you've practiced since you got married and had kids. A TIA can be your last chance for penitence. Do not ignore the sometimes subtle warning signs of a mini-stroke. Do so at your own peril – a lifetime of paralysis, diapers, frustration, depression, loss of communication, and early-onset of dementia might be at stake.

TIA: Newly Defined

TIA is no longer defined by how long symptoms last. If sudden brain-related symptoms come on *like lightning* and last usually under an hour, then experts recommend getting a CT scan, or preferably an MRI, within 24 hours. No evidence of brain damage – it *might* have been a TIA rather than a stroke. There are, of course, other ailments that can mimic a TIA or stroke and they must always be considered (see section, *Mimics of Stroke and TIA*). Another caveat: CT scans frequently do not reveal stroke damage in the early hours of a brain attack.

The Warning Signs of TIA

It is not often that people across America get a firsthand glimpse at a mini-stroke in action. That is exactly what happened as Houston Texans' football coach, Gary Kubiak, walked off the field for halftime on November 3, 2013 when he suddenly collapsed onto his knees, fell to the side, and grimaced in distress. He was whisked off on a stretcher to a local emergency room and was diagnosed as having suffered a TIA. Watch the event yourself by searching for the YouTube video.

Most common variety medical ailments get better within a few days: flu, backache, arthritis pain or bronchitis. No worries. It's all good. No doctor visit necessary. Life goes on. Not so with TIA. Symptoms may *not* be unbearable and likely will resolve quickly. These two features *usually* suggest a problem is not serious – self-limited, as doctors like to call it. *But TIA breaks this emergency care rule.* That sudden dizzy spell, or vision disturbance, or loss for words, or numb sensation in the arm or leg that comes and goes swiftly is your buzzing alarm that life-altering danger might be lurking ahead.

Sometimes learning the signs and symptoms of a TIA or stroke is simply not enough. In a widely-publicized case that can be found in a Google or YouTube search, a 49-year-old Toronto woman came to realize she must educate her doctors as well. She was evaluated at an emergency room for resolved tingling on her left side with some heaviness in her left arm. They did a basic evaluation and the brain imaging test – likely a CT scan – was normal. Home she went with advice to manage her stress by breathing deeply. Within days she experienced the same symptoms and recorded her

TIA in progress on her smartphone. Brilliant, a mini-stroke selfie! Doctors then got serious and ordered an MRI and other tests. They found the woman had serious blockages in her arteries. This is a great lesson to learn for Baby Boomers: Document your illness, if possible, to eliminate doctor diagnostic biases like a tendency to label vague symptoms as anxiety.

She was lucky not to suffer a disabling stroke, but the more concerning question is why her ER doctors did not realize her symptoms were classic for mini-stroke and treat her aggressively despite the "normal" test result? Watch the video of her experience at this link or search Google for "Woman's selfie video of stroke."

http://www.cbc.ca/news/health/stroke-diagnosis-made-through-woman-s-selfie-video-1.2677550

Common Images to Help Recall TIA and Stroke Symptoms

Symptoms usually come on like a bat out of hell – quickly, suddenly, powerfully – like a lightning bolt. The attack usually resolves in less than 60 minutes and sometimes under five minutes. Following are common stroke or TIA signs and symptoms followed by easy to remember images to use as associations. Each person can pick the images that stick in their memory for best recall.

Sign#1: Speech difficulty, drooping mouth, face numbness

IMAGES: (a) Surgeon's mask (b) Duct tape on a kidnap victim's mouth

Sign #2: Loss of vision in one eye, blurred vision, bumping into objects

IMAGES: (a) Pirate's eye patch (b) Blindfolded person playing "Pin the Tail on the Donkey" (c) Cyclops, the one-eyed monster in Greek mythology

Sign #3: Weakness, numbness, heaviness or paralysis of one arm and/or leg

IMAGES: (a) Captain Ahab's wooden leg (chewed off by Moby Dick)

(b) Captain Hook with a hook to replace his hand bitten off by a crocodile (c) "Dead-leg" numbness after sitting too long on a chair or toilet seat (d) 'Funny bone' sensation after bumping elbow

Sign #4: Severe headache

IMAGES: (a) Fouled-off baseball whacking fan in the head (b) Horror movie with axe sticking out of person's head (apologies for this one) **(c) Migraine sufferer clutching sides of head while wincing from pain**

Sign #5: Dizziness, imbalance

IMAGES: (a) Stumbling after stepping off carousel ride (b) Child twirling round and round, then stumbling about (c) Cartoon character clunked in head, stars circling around head with musical notes for dizzy feeling

Sign #6: Unexplained falls

IMAGES: (a) Slip on banana peel (b) Fall on ice while ice skating

Sign #7: Confusion, not making sense, disoriented, cannot complete or explain common adage like, "Haste makes waste."

IMAGES: (a) ? Question mark (b) "Speaking Swahili" expression for not understanding someone (c) Image of somebody standing while scratching their head

How High is Stroke Risk in Folks who Suffer a TIA?

Extremely high risk! This is particularly true in the few days after suffering a TIA. One in 20 people who have a TIA will suffer a full-blown stroke within two days. What's more, TIA sufferers have a one in four chance (25%) of being rocked by a stroke, heart attack, repeat TIA or death within 90 days! One can plainly see from these scary statistics why ignoring possibly mild TIA symptoms is not a wise approach. Identify your personal risk factors, eliminate modifiable risks, and know the signs and symptoms of TIA or stroke.

Strike Three – Stroking Out: Signs and Symptoms of the Main Event

Some folks are not lucky enough to get that precious warning called TIA. Others sadly ignore the flashing lights of mini-stroke and then suffer an irreversible brain attack. Yet others seek help appropriately but are misdiagnosed. Less typical symptoms of stroke can make the diagnosis tricky and elusive. About one-third of strokes in the back of the brain are initially misdiagnosed. What is more, a 2014 study by Dr. David Newman- Toker, a neurology researcher at Johns Hopkins Hospital, found that 13 percent of people diagnosed with a stroke were evaluated in the previous 30 days for symptoms of **headache** or **dizziness**. This suggests many stroke sufferers might have had a milder stroke or TIA misdiagnosed in the days leading up to that more serious attack.

Following are the typical as well as less common signs and symptoms of full-blown stroke. At this point, you are now "stroking out" and might be forced to face a lifetime of paralysis, loss of independence, difficulty communicating, diaper changes and memory loss. It is now Strike Three! While many stroke survivors do make excellent recoveries, there is no way to know how severe or permanent your stroke disability will be. Furthermore, recall that few truly *safe* and effective treatment options exist for brain attacks (see, Treatment section).

The Symptoms and Signs of Stroking Out

Stroke symptoms strike like lightning and are mostly the same as those experienced by TIA sufferers – except they are now *irreversible*! If you notice any of these signs in a loved one or if you personally experience any of these symptoms, CALL 911 without delay. Time wasted is brain cells lost!

- Weakness or heavy feeling in an arm, leg and/or cheek on one side of the body. Inability to raise both arms equally (arm drift), for instance.
- Severe headache, probably unlike any headache experienced in the past.
- Numbness, tingling or pain sensation on one side of the body.

- Drooping of one side of the mouth with difficulty smiling, slurred speech and possibly drooling.
- "Brain Fog" – Confusion, difficulty understanding what others say, speaking gibberish or strange-sounding speech. Less commonly, reduced consciousness. Unable to repeat a simple phrase or common expression.
- **Dizziness**, carousel-like room-spinning sensation, loss of balance, unexplained falls. Studies suggest **imbalance** to be more predictive of brain attacks. That is to say, experiencing sudden difficulty walking or being rendered unable to sit or stand upright without assistance.
- Vision disturbances: Loss of vision, blurred or double vision, bumping into objects.
- Seizures. Brain attack is the most common cause of seizures in older adults.
- Vomiting – More common in brain attack caused by bleeding into the brain.
- One recent study found that women were more likely to have **altered mental status** (change in awareness, behavior, communication, concentration, attentiveness) as the major sign of stroke.

Common signs or actions someone might observe in stroke sufferers: Unexplained fall, sudden confusion, difficulty understanding or uttering speech (mumbling or gibberish), bumping into objects, inability to fully use an arm or leg, or arm dangling limply near body.

Treatment of Stroke: Few Good Options

Clot-Busting Drugs: Miracle Treatment or Serious Danger for Stroke?

All was quiet as the healer scraped away with his instrument at the sick man's skull. The liquid anesthesia had kicked in. The healer scraped and bored harder until the instrument broke through into the brain cavity. Who was the healer? An ancient medicine man. The instrument was a bronze knife. The anesthesia was likely an alcohol-based concoction or some other mind-altering drug, if anything at all was given. The fashionable procedure: Trephination. Trephining was a widely used treatment in ancient times in which holes were scraped or drilled into the skull while the patient was awake! The procedure "cured" many serious ailments such as headaches, convulsions, insanity – or so they thought. How did it cure disease? It was believed to release evil humors or spirits. Needless to say, we no longer use this procedure as it was performed during Neolithic times 7000 years ago. It likely killed far more people than it benefitted, but seemed like the best treatment to do at the time.

Is clot-dissolving treatment for stroke a miracle cure or the modern version of trephining? Clot-busting treatment for heart attacks has shown great success. For stroke, however, which is actually comprised of several different types of brain disease, successful outcomes have proven far more controversial and elusive.

Despite clot-busting treatment recently getting the blessing of major emergency medicine organizations such as American College of Emergency Physicians, many respected emergency medicine experts argue that good reason exists for skepticism about whether clot-dissolving treatment is truly effective and safe for stroke. Many articles have been published summarizing the design flaws and possible conflicts of interest in drug company-sponsored studies with acronyms such as NINDS and ECASS. Dr Jerome Hoffman, Professor Emeritus of Emergency Medicine at UCLA Medical Center, believes the studies which formed the basis for using clot-dissolving drugs for stroke show no clear benefit, yet can be dangerous for some people. He also emphasizes in personal communication to this author (JC) that these studies had very controlled conditions yet still failed to show benefit. Imagine getting these treatments in the real-world chaos of community and teaching hospital emergency rooms! There is great risk for mistakes and possibly fatal outcomes. Newer Roto-rooter procedures in which a wire is inserted into brain arteries to physically remove blood clots have shown mixed results in the limited studies completed to date.

Some skeptical experts do believe certain patients can benefit from clot-busting treatment. Dr. David Newman-Toker, Assistant Professor of

Neurology at Johns Hopkins Hospital and a stroke expert, said in a personal communication to this author (JC):

If I were a patient with weakness on one side (of the body) and difficulty speaking, I would want to receive a clot-busting drug.

Clot-dissolving treatment for strokes remains a hotly debated topic with many emergency room physicians reluctant to offer this risky treatment they believe is not yet proven as safe and effective. Interestingly, equal numbers of emergency room doctors are sued for *not* offering this treatment as are sued for complications of administering the medication.

Reasons *Not* to Accept Risky or Invasive Stroke Treatments

1. *Natural History of Stroke Recovery*: It was not long ago, perhaps 20 years, when stroke sufferers who arrived in the emergency room were rolled into a quiet corner to allow the stroke to run its course. Virtually nothing could be done. A dramatically high blood pressure would warrant some medication, a quick prayer, and that was about all doctors had to offer. Yet many surviving stroke victims made significant recoveries. The Copenhagen Stroke Study found that after stroke rehabilitation, over three-fourths of sufferers had no deficit or only mild residual deficits from the stroke. A more recent analysis in the journal *Clinical Rehabilitation* found that almost three-fourths of stroke patients who showed some hand paralysis recovery by four weeks had a good to full recovery. Hand use recovery tends to lag behind recovery of leg function and more severe paralysis at stroke onset is a bad omen for final recovery. A 1988 study by Bonita published in the journal *Stroke* found that after 6 months, 76 percent of stroke survivors with motor function loss had mild or no remaining disability. It is noteworthy that improvement in loss of speech (aphasia) with clot-dissolving drugs is *no better* than natural recovery rates, one recent study found (Maas J Stroke Cerebrovasc Dis, July 2012). In brief summary, many stroke sufferers who survive make excellent functional recoveries even *without* any aggressive or risky treatments during the stroke.
2. Eleven of 13 large studies on clot-dissolving treatment for stroke

showed poor results and great risk yet the negative studies tend to be ignored. Even the major "positive" NINDS studies have been found to have many concerning flaws by medical experts such as Dr. Jerome Hoffman.

3. Emergency medicine medical organizations such as the American Academy of Emergency Medicine (AAEM) and the Canadian Academy of Emergency Medicine have for years been reluctant to endorse clot-busting treatment for acute stroke. In fact, the AAEM patient education tool on tPA for stroke states as of the date of this writing, "Several studies suggested (that) treatment with clot-dissolving medications increases the number of patients who die following a stroke."

4. Studies tend to show that people with the most severe strokes who would derive the most potential benefit from treatment with clot-dissolving drugs or brain artery Roto-rooter procedures are at *greatest* risk for the most serious complications such as bleeding into the brain. Older folks tend to be at higher risk from clot-busting drug complications as well.

5. Clot-busting treatments must be given as early as possible to derive any purported benefit at all – ideally within 90 minutes of first stroke symptoms. This requires immediate identification of stroke by the patient, family or friend, followed by prompt ambulance transport to an emergency room. Speedy diagnosis usually with a less accurate CT scan, sometimes an MRI, must ensue. All these steps take time. What's more, diagnosis can be tricky because many other illnesses can mimic a stroke or TIA. You would not want to get risky clot-dissolving treatment for an ailment that turns out *not* to be a stroke. Doctors would have to rush to give you this treatment in a chaotic emergency room without time for a thorough evaluation or confident diagnosis. It would be ideal for a neurologist to consult and confirm the diagnosis and benefits of aggressive treatment. But there is no time for that as those precious 90 minutes are quickly ticking away. Risks of rushing the stroke diagnosis may outweigh any possible treatment benefits if it turns out to be a stroke. Furthermore, recent studies done in Berlin,

Germany administered clot-busting drugs in a CT-scan-equipped ambulance! As if the emergency room is not chaotic enough and a worrisome setup for errors.

6. *Stroke Mimics*: Doctors can easily be fooled by many medical problems that mimic a stroke or TIA but have completely different causes. Seizure, low blood sugar and electrolyte abnormalities are just a few examples of pitfalls in which, in their rush to give clot-busting drug treatment promptly, might mistakenly administer this risky drug to someone who suffers a mimic illness.
7. *Reperfusion Injury*: A nutrient-carrying artery gets plugged up to cause a stroke. The clot-dissolving drug unclogs the artery and blood is again flowing freely. Problem solved, right? Patient gets better fast? Not so simple. All those toxins and inflammation cells that built up at the blockage site now flood through. Other unknown factors may also contribute to compound cell injury and cell death even after the blockage is opened. Don't you wish strokes worked simply like when Drano unclogs a pipe? What's more, the toxin-rich blood that floods into the injured area of the brain can increase chances for brain hemorrhage, another serious complication.
8. *Micro-hemorrhages*: Small areas of brain bleeding have been found on MRI to be fairly common in older adults, those with high blood pressure, smokers, and in folks who have previously suffered a stroke. One general population study found tiny brain micro-bleeds in 6.5 percent of people 45-50 years old and as high as 35 percent of folks over 80 years of age. Moreover, about one-fourth of those people who suffer an ischemic stroke are found to have tiny brain bleeds that might portend a higher risk of catastrophic bleeding if given clot-dissolving treatment.

Is clot-dissolving treatment for stroke a modern-day trephining treatment that will someday prove to be as barbaric and dangerous as when ancient medicine men drilled holes into skulls to cure headaches and seizures? For now, a quick yet thorough discussion between family members and doctors must take place to determine if that stroke sufferer wants a doctor to tinker with his or her brain under rushed and chaotic conditions, using treatments that remain risky and controversial. Most importantly, learn to recognize signs and symptoms of brain attack, cut through the denial, and CALL 911 or have someone drive you to an emergency room quickly as possible. If you are rapidly diagnosed as suffering a stroke, you will at least have options to accept or reject riskier treatments.

What Can Emergency Room Stroke Centers Offer?

Some emergency rooms offer special areas that treat only suspected stroke or TIA sufferers. Identifying a subtle TIA, however, is very difficult in triage so many actual mini-stroke victims will wind up in the main emergency department anyway. The goal is to streamline diagnosis and treatment similar to chest pain units for heart attacks. Following is a list of theoretical benefits and caveats of stroke center treatment:

1. tPA clot dissolving treatment: Based on 2011 Medicare claims data, only about four percent of stroke sufferers received clot-dissolving drug treatment.
2. Mechanically opening the plugged brain artery like stent placement with heart attack, known as endovascular therapy: Studies thus far show spotty but questionable benefit and great risk for invasive procedures over standard treatments. One hope for invasive treatments is that special MRI or CT scan imaging can identify brain cells that are nutrient-starved but not yet dead. People with larger areas of still-living brain tissue were presumed to be better candidates for invasively unclogging the stroke artery with Roto-rooter-like devices. Studies to date have been mixed at best. Still so much we do not understand about the brain!
3. Experimental trials of many new and varied approaches to stroke treatment: For instance, several recent studies published in the *New England Journal of Medicine* have found "stent retriever" devices successful at mechanically removing blood clots from larger brain arteries. Will this technique alter the balance of risk versus benefit for invasive stroke treatments? Time will surely sort this out.
4. Special training: Perhaps prompt assessment by doctors who are more familiar with stroke-related disease and subtleties of TIA.

5. Active supportive care from specially-trained nurses and aids.

Are there Clear Benefits to Stroke Treatment at a Stroke Center?

Dr. Jerome Hoffman, Emergency Medicine Professor at UCLA Medical Center, explains that stroke center treatment benefits are currently purely anecdotal. No objective studies show clear benefit in outcomes at stroke centers versus regular ER care. Some possible explanations for seemingly better stroke center care include doctors and nurses paying closer attention to the stroke patient, doctors who are familiar with the diseases that mimic a stroke, perhaps more immediate availability of imaging tests with fewer delays than in a community hospital, and possibly less chaos in a stroke center relative to a general emergency department. Excellent rehabilitation and anticipation of potential complications might also contribute to better results at stroke centers.

The disadvantages rest primarily in risk from getting more invasive or experimental treatments. Do you want some doctor experimenting with or tinkering with your brain? Any of these less proven stroke treatments are at best controversial, possibly helpful in some patients, but highly risky. If things do not go well with invasive brain treatments, the consequence may well be death. Are these treatments worth taking? Perhaps if a stroke sufferer quickly has full paralysis of an arm and leg and full loss of speech that seems to be progressing and not improving by the time diagnosis is complete, then consideration of aggressive stroke treatment might be worth the risks. A reminder: Many stroke sufferers show excellent recovery in the weeks following stroke even without risking invasive treatments. Each person must get a detailed explanation of risks versus benefits and quickly decide if simple and safer treatment is prudent rather than high-stakes Roto-rooter procedures on the brain. Just because we *can* do these procedures, does not mean it is worth the potential dangers.

A Few Tips and Reminders

- In the emergency room, doctors might not take you seriously if you walk in feeling fine and tell them you "got dizzy" for a few minutes. Busy ER staff might well mistakenly conclude you had common variety vertigo. They might order a less accurate brain

CT scan and send you on your way. It seems you may be better off avoiding that false reassurance and high out-of-pocket cost. Instead, consider an urgent visit to see your doctor in the office within about 24 hours. Discuss your concerns about TIA and stroke, mention your known risk factors, and suggest you would like a thorough evaluation. Consider daily low-dose aspirin treatment to reduce risk of recurrent events. A complete work up might include brain MRI and possibly MRA (chemical angiogram) within 24 hrs, ultrasound of the carotid (neck) and brain arteries, electrocardiogram and 24-hour heart monitor to check for atrial fibrillation, and blood tests such as lipids, liver enzymes, glucose, C-Reactive Protein, hemoglobin A1c to screen for diabetes, and routine blood tests. An echocardiogram of the heart and sonogram of the liver might offer useful information as well, if necessary.

- Never forget that 80 percent of strokes are *preventable*, according to the American Stroke Association.
- Preventing brain attacks *before* they occur is surely more effective and safe than currently available, sometimes hotly debated, stroke therapies.
- Discuss with your doctor whether you should take low-dose aspirin for a few weeks after suffering from a nasty winter respiratory infection or a bout of shingles. Stroke risk has been found to rise after significant infections such as flu, bronchitis or shingles.
- Discuss with your doctor whether risks outweigh benefits for taking low-dose aspirin after suffering from a possible TIA that is never confidently confirmed or negated.
- CT scan of the brain is a far less accurate test to diagnose TIA or mild stroke compared with MRI. This is especially true in the first few hours after symptoms begin. Take the result with a grain of salt if told "everything is okay on the CT scan."
- Five factors associated with **higher risk** for stroke within 90 days after suffering a TIA (mini-stroke):
    * Age over 60
    * TIA symptoms lasting more than 10 minutes

* Arm or leg weakness on one side of the body
* Speech impairment during TIA
* Having diabetes mellitus

Stroke Quiz – Don't Take it at Your Own Risk

Will you be able recognize a stroke?

Do you have the facts to identify a brain attack or TIA in progress? Time wasted might mean millions more dead brain cells. Let us see how well you do:

1. Name three signs (what is observed) or symptoms (what is felt) of a stroke.

____

____

2. Name three signs or symptoms of a TIA or mini-stroke.

____

____

3. What are three *risk factors* for a stroke?

____

____

4. Which of the following is *most* likely to be directly associated with a stroke or TIA?

   a. Degree of dizziness

   b. Severe fatigue

   c. Feeling faint

   d. Very abrupt onset of symptoms

5. Which of the following is *most* likely to be directly associated with a stroke or TIA?

   a. Loss of consciousness

   b. Tingling in both hands

   c. Sudden weakness or tingling on one side of the body

   d. Cramping or weakness in both legs

6. Why is it so important to find out if rapid onset brain-related symptoms that come and go within minutes was likely or unlikely to be a mini-stroke (TIA)?

Come back to these questions after you have reread the chapter on stroke. You can find the answers to these questions on the book website at **http://www.endlessknotpress.com/category/boomer-the-book/**

IV. RED FLAGS: HOW CAREGIVERS CAN IDENTIFY ILLNESS IN FRAIL ELDERS BEFORE CALAMITY STRIKES

The Golden 72 Hours: Identifying and Treating Illness *before* the Crisis

If you are a caregiver for frail elders, be sure to read the chapter on dangers of hospitalization. Once you have read that eye-opening chapter you will be convinced that seniors should avoid the hospital, if possible. How can you help to prevent medical crises that require hospital transfer? The elderly typically show *gradual deterioration* from illness that ultimately unravels into a life or death calamity. In truth, one cannot always prevent medical calamity. Doctors have not yet solved human mortality, frailty and vulnerability. Old folks with serious chronic ailments suffer health catastrophes such as heart attacks or strokes or sepsis and many other life-threatening crises. Yet there are many instances in which less serious, more subtle ailments can be identified *early* and treated promptly and aggressively. Identifying and treating illness early can help to avoid many ER visits and hospitalizations. You, the caregiver, are on the front lines of care and should be properly informed to achieve this goal. Once the ailment is identified, your task is to do common sense actions that can slow deterioration – until professional medical help arrives. Why is this so vital? Simply put, the hospital is the worst place to be if you are old and sick – as long as the illness is *not* immediately life-threatening. Crises that imminently threaten life or limb surely warrant hospitalization. If, on the other hand, a senior is nearing the end of life, hospice-based comfort or palliative care might be most appropriate rather than subjecting these delicate seniors to havoc, discomfort, confusion and risks of acute hospitalization and the tests and procedures that go with it (see also, Last Wishes Planning: Don't Worry, Die Happy chapter).

Caregivers must have the proper tools of the trade and set up in advance a few key systems and processes:

1. Develop a good relationship and close communication capabilities with a trusted and respected home-visiting medical practice or office-based provider. The home-visiting doctor or nurse practitioner must be available for urgent visits on the same day or next day, not just routine monthly visits. For office-based providers, they

must be willing to work with the caregiver through phone calls and faxed orders since it is impractical to transport frail, sick older adults to an office for every health concern.

2. Put together an advance preferred plan for each frail older adult should acute illness strike. Does he or she want aggressive medical care at the hospital? Or is that senior near the end of life and prefers only comfort care and perhaps hospice services? These details should be worked out immediately with family, the resident and healthcare provider to assure each person receives the type of care desired. Development of an advance directive plan of care can be helpful in addressing these key care issues (see also, Last Wishes Planning: Don't Worry, Die Happy chapter).
3. Have an in-depth medication discussion with the primary care provider. Learn which medications should be reduced or held for various common problems as discussed below. For older folks, less is usually better with regard to medication.
4. Establish a custom-tailored routine for simple exercises for every older adult. It can be walking, stationary cycling, resistance against weights or an elastic band. Leg and arm lifts and range of motion exercises in bed or a chair can be helpful for even the most infirm folks. More muscle equals more independence and function and better medication metabolism.
5. Put together an individualized nutrition and food plan for each older adult. Favorite foods. Ethnic preferences. Palatable textures. Social eating environment. Accommodate for chewing and swallowing difficulties. Frequent healthy snacks several times a day may be necessary for older folks who typically cannot eat larger meals.

Tools of the Trade

As a caregiver on the front lines of care, paid or unpaid, you must be fitted with the proper tools of the trade if you are going to succeed. Car mechanics have their large red toolboxes filled to the brim. Plumbers have their trucks packed with copper pipes, oversized wrenches and coiled snakes. Doctors have their not-so-little-anymore doctors' bags carefully stocked with indispensible medical tools. Selfless caretakers must also be proactive and properly prepared for the saintly task of caring for the needy and infirm. Plan wisely and in advance by researching and purchasing crucial tools of the care-giving trade. If a caretaker is going to successfully identify illness early, certain procedures should be followed to monitor seniors.

Since many older folks in assisted living these days are infirm and needy enough to be in a skilled nursing facility, it is time for a culture change. While maintaining the at-home feel so important to the assisted living and adult care home crowd, there must be some "medicalization" of care homes. Vital signs should be carefully monitored for these folks as in a skilled facility. Ideally, a home-visiting provider should oversee care in the facility or home. These procedures will require a well-stocked "Caregiver Toolbox." Here is what should be kept in it:

The Caregiver Toolbox

- **Stethoscope**: Use a decent quality stethoscope (or 'Adscope') to hear breath sounds and the heartbeat. Littman stethoscopes and ADC Adscopes are generally a good bet. Those five and ten dollar stethoscopes with pretty colors – probably a waste of money. Do some research online and expect to pay between 50 and 100 dollars for a stethoscope that works well and allows the user to hear well the heart rhythm and rate, lung sounds, and even steady, low-level intestinal gurgling to be sure the intestinal factory is working okay inside the abdomen.
- **Pulse Oximeter**: A finger oximeter to measure blood oxygen levels is a vital tool for seniors who are experiencing difficulty breathing, wheezing, confusion, lethargy or coughing. An oxygen saturation level below 90 percent, or much lower than their usual level, suggests trouble is brewing and warrants an urgent doctor visit in the home, if available. These nifty gadgets used to cost $250 for a quality oximeter. Many fine finger oximeters can now be purchased online for 30 to 75 dollars. Just read online reviews about any device you plan to buy. Note: Oximeters are sensitive to room lighting and should be shielded from excess ambient lighting for more accurate results.
- **Blood Pressure Cuff**: A digital *arm* cuff is preferable to a wrist

device, generally speaking. Once again, read online reviews for better quality products. Quality cuffs can run 50 to 100 dollars. It is also wise to use the device when a doctor or nurse measures the person's blood pressure to compare your device for accuracy. Also check blood pressure on both left and right arms for baseline measurement and to check for large differences between sides. Always measure blood pressure in the elderly when sitting AND standing, supported if necessary. Blood pressure can drop significantly when standing, a common problem called orthostatic hypotension which can cause dizziness, weakness or falls. For bedridden or infirm folks, check the pressure when lying back and with legs dangling off the side of the bed. A drop in pressure sitting to standing of 20 mm Hg systolic or 10 mm Hg diastolic should be reported to the provider promptly.

- **Sitting Weight Scale**: Monitoring for daily or weekly weight changes is crucial in caring for the elderly and in early recognition of simmering sicknesses such as heart failure (fluid backed up in the lungs). Heart failure causes a gradual buildup of fluid in the body, causing weight gain. The ankles may swell but not always. Breathing becomes more labored, especially with simple activities. Lying down flat also can precipitate severe breathing distress in someone who has worsening heart failure. Monthly or weekly weight measurement can also be useful in monitoring for failure to thrive or hidden cancer in the elderly. Significant weight loss (10 percent of body weight) can qualify a senior for hospice services as well. Since many frail elderly cannot stand steadily on a scale, a sitting scale can be valuable. Most of these scales are prohibitively pricey but a search online for a used scale can strike gold. Two options for a new sitting scale include the skimpier Health-O-Meter Portable Seat Scale, 250 lb Capacity, which retails for about 100 dollars and the Detecto 475 Mechanical Medical Chair Scale, 350 lb capacity, which has an actual seat but retails for about 500 dollars. Either way, these can be a useful investment for caregivers. Digital standing scales can sometimes be difficult to use in older folks so old fashioned meter scales might be a better choice.
- **Glucometer:** Every care home for frail elders should have a

glucometer available to check the blood sugar of diabetics and any person who passes out or is suddenly lethargic, weak, sweaty or shaky. When a home health nurse visits, have the nurse instruct you on proper blood sugar fingerstick technique. Another option: a doctor can order diabetes education by a trained educator. Free glucometers are sometimes obtainable, or save an old one to use as backup. Remember to test any glucometer with the test solution that is included with the device. Caveat: When logging daily blood sugars, always tell the provider about a *new pattern* of several low sugars under 85 or very high levels above 300. Medication and diet adjustments should be made.

- **Hand Grip-Strength Dynamometer:** These gadgets can be purchased for 20 to 40 dollars and can serve to measure increasing weakness in a frail senior. The dynamometer is not as important as the other tools of the trade since most caregivers have a keen awareness of when someone is weaker than usual. Seniors usually lose some function capability when too weak to walk, stand or give support with transfers. Having an objective strength measure or number by using this gizmo can be helpful for early detection of health status changes.
- **Urine pH Test Strips:** This is something you as caregiver probably never tried. Testing urine acidity versus alkalinity can give key information for caregivers in trying to prevent urinary tract infections. Many bacteria thrive in alkaline conditions. In addition, kidney stones are more likely to form with acid urine: orange juice, lemon or lime added to the diet can help alkalinize (higher pH) urine and reduce kidney stone formation. These pH strips for urine can be ordered online for less than 15 dollars per large pack. See Urinary Tract Infection section below for additional details.
- **Log Sheets to Monitor Vital Signs:** It is crucial to watch for changes in a senior's baseline vital signs which could signal an early clue that illness is brewing. This practice can no longer be limited to hospitals and skilled facilities. Key vital signs are heart rate (and rhythm – regular or irregular beat), blood pressure (too high or too low or significant change from baseline), breathing rate and quality

(labored, wheezy or comfortable), and weight. For diabetics, blood sugar can be logged as well. When a significant pneumonia or urinary infection is brewing, for instance, a diabetic's blood sugars may bump higher. All people may show an increase in heart rate from baseline due to breathing deterioration, infection, fever or dehydration. Accelerated heart rate can be the earliest sign of simmering sickness. A noticeably lower blood pressure from baseline can also indicate dehydration or dreaded sepsis (blood infection). Log sheets can be printed from word processing software using a 'table' insertion of rows and columns that fits the size of a standard sheet of paper.

- **Thermometer:** Fever response is frequently blunted or absent in the elderly even with serious illnesses that would have younger adults burning up. Forehead (temporal artery), mouth (oral) and armpit (axillary) temperature measurements can be inconsistent or inaccurate as well. For instance, temporal artery measurements can be affected by sweating which cools the skin. Rectal temperature measurement can be impractical in sick elders, requires a few minutes for accurate readings, and can have its own inconsistencies. Tympanic (ear) temperatures are likely most convenient in older adults since measurement takes a few seconds. An ear temperature probe measures heat given off by the eardrum, which shares blood supply with the temperature-regulating center in the brain. However, large earwax build up could affect accuracy, although some manufacturer information claims wax does *not* affect accuracy. Common sense, however, says otherwise. Some manufacturers claim that the ear measurement is more accurate than the forehead device. As hazy as temperature measurement accuracy can be, two key points seem clear based upon the medical research literature: First, older folks tend to have a *lower* temperature baseline. Caregivers should take several temperature measurements over a couple of weeks using a quality tympanic scanner. Record the average of those few readings as the baseline temperature. Research has found that an ear temperature of about 99 degrees (37 degrees Celsius) is the upper limit of normal for older folks (100.3 degrees Fahrenheit is upper limit for younger adults). Second, a *rise* of 1.3

to 1.5 degrees above that person's *baseline* temperature can be considered a fever. Three tympanic temperature measurements done over several hours and averaged out would be best to confirm presence of fever. All accuracy bets might be off, however, if the ear canal is fully occluded with wax, a common problem in older folks. This is why doctors focus less on fever in the elderly and look for changes in condition as a more accurate measure of infection or other illness. If funds are available, using both a temporal artery and tympanic device to compare consistency of measurements might be useful. These fancy digital thermometers can cost up to $50 each. Just to reiterate, despite accuracy concerns with many temperature devices, the key is to establish a *baseline* 'normal' temperature for each person by taking several measurements at different times over a few days when the person is feeling fine. Use the same device for all measurements and that average is the 'normal' baseline. When sickness strikes, take two or three temperature measurements over a couple hours with the same device. If the average temperature is more than 1.3 to 1.5 degrees *above* baseline then that should be considered a true fever.

Action-Reaction Approach - Common Sense Caring

It is hard to make care decisions while lacking special medical knowledge and training, and without a fancy, framed diploma hanging on the wall. Yet caregivers are tasked with steep responsibility for the well-being of sickly residents. Do not despair. Much of basic medical decision-making made by healthcare providers is common sense, not rocket science. Use what I call the "Action-Reaction Approach" to managing health issues among sick older folks and you will do right by those who depend upon you, until a trusted medical professional arrives. The concept is simple: When a problem arises do the *opposite* or simply what makes sense. It is exactly what any competent medical professional would recommend. Then you can notify the provider about the temporary changes you made until help arrives. Following are some common issues that arise with older folks and the response (reaction) you should have, like a reflex or law of physics:

► **Loss of Appetite or Nausea** – Avoid heavy, spicy or acidy foods. Hold off on dispensing nonessential pills. Offer fluids with electrolytes (*not* only plain water) and bland foods like yogurt, pudding, gelatin dessert, chicken broth or similar clear soups, banana, toast, or other favorite but bland foods. Ask the doctor in advance what new drugs or those on the medication list are likely to affect appetite or cause stomach upset. Consider holding those medications until the provider can do an evaluation. Common offender drugs include aspirin or ibuprofen, many antibiotics, and memory drugs. If vomiting occurs, hold all nonessential drugs and supplements as planned in advance in discussions with the provider. It is wise to mark each medication with doctor guidance as either "essential" or "non-essential." Any noticeable drop in food or fluid intake for even a day or two, for instance, should reflexively lead to holding off on diuretic drugs such as lasix, bumex, HCTZ, maxzide, metolazone or spironolactone. Work out a plan in advance with the primary provider as to how to best approach this.

► **Lethargy, Loss of Functional Ability or Sleeps all Day** – If this problem is new, that person should get a prompt medical evaluation, preferably from a visiting doctor or nurse practitioner. It is common for old folks to have vague medical complaints while dropping a notch on the function scale. Losing ability to walk, self-toilet, self-feed, or assist with transfers into the bed or chair are common function losses that can signal serious illness is brewing. In the meanwhile, consider if there are any changes in condition to suggest a urine or lung infection. Know in advance which medications can cause drowsiness or weakness or search the internet for that information. Let the doctor know you are holding off on giving those medications if the person is already overly tired, sleepy or weak. Common culprit drugs that cause drowsiness include sleeping pills, narcotic pain pills, seizure or mood-stabilizer drugs, muscle relaxants, psychiatric drugs, and off-the-shelf antihistamines or multi-symptom cold remedies. Weakness can be caused by low blood pressure, dehydration, infection, low blood sugar, overly-sedating medications, stroke, heart attack and a thousand other medical problems.

► **Up Much of the Night** – Avoid daytime napping. Encourage daytime exercises such as walking around the house, garden, facility or neighborhood, with assistance as needed. Limit caffeinated drinks such as coffee, tea, soda pop or energy drinks. Ask the doctor if any medications might be contributing to insomnia. Do you suspect a medical problem is contributing to insomnia such as sundowning, pain, coughing, trouble breathing, bad dreams or anxiety, or waking up many times to urinate? Relay that information to the doctor.

▶ **High Blood Pressure** – If someone you are caring for has experienced sharp rises in blood pressure, you should devise a plan with the primary care provider to have an extra blood pressure medication available on an as needed basis. Another option is to give an extra dose of a drug that person already takes, if the blood pressure shoots above a specified level. Generally speaking, a blood pressure of about 150-160/90 or less in an older adult who is feeling fine does not necessarily require any treatment. Some old folks function better when their pressure is 170 systolic (top number) than when it is treated down to 120. This "perfect" pressure of 120, at times, can cause weakness and dizziness in the elderly. In those who have had strokes, a pressure below 140/85 is safer; however, each patient requires an individualized approach depending on their overall condition, other medical ailments, medication tolerance, and quality of life preferences.

▶ **Low Blood Pressure** – Several studies have confirmed that a blood pressure that drops too low can increase death rates in older folks. The diastolic pressure (bottom number) is what forces blood into the heart-nourishing arteries during heartbeat relaxation (diastole). If the pressure is too low, the heart could be deprived of needed blood and oxygen, leading to heart troubles. Experts recommend the diastolic blood pressure ideally remain between 70 and 80 mm Hg. Diastolic pressure under 60 mm Hg should prompt consideration of medication reduction and perhaps added salt to the diet. If the person is unusually weak or gets woozy standing or sitting up then a pressure below 65-70 mm Hg may be too low. Simple actions to take: reduce the dosage of a blood pressure medication as recommended by the healthcare provider; or hold the next dose of that pressure-lowering drug until you get specific advice from a provider; one can also add salt to the diet and increase fluids (not just water) to boost the blood pressure.

▶ **Rapid or Slow Heart Rate** – Heart rate is best measured by using a quality stethoscope to listen to the left side of the chest. This will get you an "apical" heart rate, meaning directly from the heart. Why not just feel the wrist pulse? Not all heart beats are transmitted to the wrist in folks with atrial fibrillation, meaning the heart can at times be racing with an irregular rhythm of 140 but the wrist pulse will measure only about 70 to

80 beats per minute. Count every beat of the heart using a stethoscope for a timed 30 seconds, then multiply that counted number by two. That gives you a more accurate apical heart rate. For normal rhythm hearts, a finger pulse oximeter measures heart rate accurately and easily. Note whether the rhythm of the heart beat is regular and predictable or totally irregular and all over the place. A significant change in heart rate above or below the baseline recorded rate that persists with a few measurements over six to twelve hours suggests a problem such as a heart arrhythmia, breathing trouble, infection, dehydration, fever or thyroid excess. A very slow heart rate can be caused by too much medication (atenolol, metoprolol, carvedilol, verapamil, diltiazem most common) or primary heart problems. Holding doses of heart-slowing medication like metoprolol or atenolol can help a slow heart rate. Rapid heart rates can be more complicated. Both conditions warrant a call to the primary care provider or cardiologist, especially if the person complains of chest pain, breathing difficulty, or feeling unusually weak, sleepy or dizzy. Deviations in heart rate from someone's baseline are most useful; however, as a general rule a heart rate under 50 to 55 beats per minute warrants careful attention and a prompt medical evaluation if the person feels unwell with that low heart rate. On the high end, over 100 beats per minute is surely problematic but a persistent change from a baseline of 60, up to 85 beats per minute, for example, would be quite worrisome as well.

▶ **Diarrhea or Loose, Frequent Bowel Movements** – If the 'runs' come, hold any recently added medications with the doctor's permission. Stop stool softeners and laxatives until the bowels return toward regular routine. Avoid dairy foods except cultured yogurt since diarrhea can cause temporary lactose intolerance. Offer a 'BRAT' diet which includes bananas, rice, apple sauce and toast. Chicken broth with rice or miso soup can be good options as well. Use of constipating medications like Imodium, Lomotil and Kaopectate can be helpful if the primary care provider has evaluated the senior and recommends as needed use. Avoid caffeine which stimulates the intestines. Be alert for C. Difficile diarrhea when many watery and extremely foul smelling movements occur daily, particularly in those who were in a hospital or skilled facility or who received antibiotics within the past few weeks.

▶ **Constipation** – Since constipation is the "default setting" in older folks,

I will not go into depth on this topic now except to recommend dietary measures first. Oatmeal, prunes, dates, prune juice, beets and raisins are healthy and can stimulate regular bowel movements. Caffeine could be helpful in theory since it stimulates the intestines. Many medications can add to constipation problems such as narcotic pain relievers, overactive bladder drugs, and certain blood pressure medications. Check with the doctor if any medications might be stopping things up.

▶ **Low Blood Sugar** – How do you know if the blood sugar level drops low? Common signs are lethargy, confusion, weakness, shakiness, profuse sweating, blurred vision, racing heart, dizziness, headache and even passing out. Treatment for suspected or confirmed low blood sugar is to use a quickly absorbing sugar source such as a tablespoon of sugar or honey under the tongue or a glucose gel, or *sips* of one-third cup of sweet juice. After the sugar level improves, slowly-absorbing sugar sources can help prevent a delayed drop in blood sugar level by offering milk, eating half a slice of bread, or some nuts, for instance. If sugar logs show more than one glucose (sugar) value under 75-80 then healthy snack frequency must be increased or medication dose (pills or insulin) should be reduced promptly based upon doctor advice – before critically low sugar level lands the senior in the emergency room.

▶ **High Blood Sugar** – Frail older diabetics generally should be satisfied if their blood sugar stays between 100 and 180. Their life expectancy is not long so future diabetes complications are not as concerning. Too low values (below 75-80) can be worse than too high (200 level) in these folks. Ask the healthcare provider at what high level of blood sugar to be worried. One isolated high value over 300 is not typically a problem; several consistently high values might suggest dehydration or infection or diabetes gone out of control.

▶ **Too Many Meds!** – Any time an older adult has a med list longer than 4 or 5 drugs, be sure the primary care provider regularly tries to reduce a dose or stop a medication. This is ever more important when a senior develops loss of appetite or vague weakness or loss of interest in activities they once enjoyed. Weight and muscle loss, dehydration, heart failure or reduced kidney function can lead to serious side effects on a drug regimen that person once tolerated well. Sometimes it is simply a domino effect with just one extra drug leading to drug-drug or drug-disease interaction which triggers overall health decline. You, as frontline caregiver, must be the advocate for older folks who are over-medicated. Why all the fuss about medication? Drugs are a common cause in older folks for falls, injuries and emergency room visits due to bad reactions. Each medication deserves careful consideration of benefits versus risks in older adults. Reminder: Medications can harm as well as help older folks.

Special Health Concerns in Older Folks

Dehydration

When an older adult is rushed to an emergency room for dehydration it is a common but dreaded event. Dehydration in older folks is often preventable and some official agencies consider this a sign of less than adequate care.

Older folks are actually quite susceptible to dehydration. As fat replaces muscle in an aging body, there is less total body water present. The elderly also have a reduced thirst sensation and their worn-out kidneys cannot efficiently conserve water when it is scarce. Throw in the following risk factors and you have a recipe for an ambulance ride to the emergency room:

- Mobility limitations, paralysis, arthritic hands, bedridden so cannot seek out fluids
- Memory loss or communication difficulty
- Depression with accompanying loss of appetite, swallowing trouble, apathy
- Multiple chronic diseases and many medications, all of which ruin the appetite
- Fear of having an accident if cannot get to the bathroom in time after drinking
- Uncontrolled diabetes, with excess sugar spillage having a diuretic effect
- Dehydrating medications such as diuretics (water pills) and laxatives

- Drying drugs like Benadryl, overactive bladder and irritable bowel medications, and antipsychotic drugs
- Diarrhea or vomiting
- Salt or fluid restriction due to heart failure, kidney failure, high blood pressure
- Excessive heat or dryness outdoors or inside, fever from infection
- Too few caregivers for many seniors, or older folks who do not want to be a bother so they avoid asking for help with drinks or food
- Anorexia of Aging – the gradual decline in appetite and food intake as we age
- Social concerns such as inability to afford enough food and beverages or inability to shop for or prepare food and drinks

To make matters worse, dehydration predisposes folks to constipation, kidney stones, blood clots, dizziness, low blood pressure, weakness, falls, confusion, and perhaps urine and lung infections. The typical signs of dehydration such as dry mouth, sunken eyes, reduced sweat, less urine output and less supple skin are *not* reliable or practical dehydration indicators in the elderly. What are some ways to detect impending dehydration in older folks? Consistent intake of *less than* 50 percent of meals puts seniors at great risk. Reduced urine output from baseline could be the best indicator that trouble is brewing but it is difficult to monitor carefully in older folks. An increased heart rate above that person's baseline is an early body response to reduced fluid in blood vessels, but heartbeat-slowing medications like metoprolol or diltiazem can blunt this response; a drop in usual blood pressure levels follows later. Lack of armpit moisture can be a clue as can a persistently darker shade of urine similar to tea-color. A dry tongue with grooves along the length of the tongue can also signal fluid and electrolyte deficiency.

If a senior loses more than two pounds in a day, that can be measurement error, or if accurate, a reflection of under-hydration. Another weight guideline for dehydration is loss of 3 percent of body weight in a short time frame. A useful general rule of thumb is the following: just over two pounds of weight (one kilogram) equals about one liter of fluid.

Proactive Prevention Strategies

- Here again, baseline vital sign monitoring is crucial. Increased heart rate, drop in blood pressure, sudden weight changes using a consistent weighing method (clothes on or off, shoes on or not, same scale on a hard floor surface).
- Urine output is hard to monitor outside a hospital setting unless a bladder catheter is in place. Other approaches caregivers can use include tracking someone's average number of brief changes for those who are incontinent, or average number of bathroom trips a senior typically makes during the day or night. These are, of course, rough estimates yet can be helpful in sounding a dehydration alarm, so to speak.
- Avoid caffeinated beverages, alcohol, and high protein drinks in those at risk for dehydration. These can promote loss of fluids.
- Have the doctor reduce diuretic dosages, if possible, or discontinue nonessential diuretics such as prescriptions for leg swelling only. Cut back on laxatives if bowel movements are loose or frequent. Minimize drying 'anticholinergic' drugs such as older antihistamines, overactive bladder prescriptions, anti-seizure drugs, and irritable bowel remedies.
- Serve favorite, healthy drinks with flavor and variety. Keep a covered cup with a large handle available near older folks so they can take sips throughout the day. Many will need reminders to drink often.
- Do *not* limit drinks to plain water. Many people find water tasteless and will not drink as much if taste buds are not stimulated. Furthermore, bottled or filtered water has virtually no electrolytes (salts) in it. A few fine options for creative hydration with variety: coconut or soy or almond milk; decaf tea; mineral drinks with high levels of magnesium, sodium and potassium (for instance, Apollinaris, Gerolsteiner, San Pellegrino); popular sports drinks; flavored water; tomato or fruit juices (straight up or diluted half water); and chicken broth or miso soup. Other options: water with lemon or cucumber. Avoid drinks that are too cold or too hot that might be unpalatable to some folks. Ice pops made from frozen

juice or sports drinks can be refreshing for some people and can be helpful for those with swallowing difficulty.

- Consider adding salt and spices to chicken broth or other soups. These add flavor and stimulate thirst.
- Room temperature and clothing worn by seniors can contribute to fluid and salt loss from sweating. Is the heat on too high and dry during cold winter months? Does the sun shine through the open window and quickly heat up a senior's room? The elderly usually feel cold and might dress in several layers even when it is warm outside or inside. This can increase sweating and cause excess fluid and salt losses. Fans can help cool rooms efficiently and closed window shades insulate against direct sunlight.
- Have older folks drink a little extra fluid when taking medications and brushing their teeth.
- Try getting older adults to eat and drink more in the *morning* since studies have found many older folks take in more food or drinks during the early hours of the day. Taking in extra liquids during daylight hours also helps avoid excessive urination during sleep.
- The elderly should be sipping small amounts of fluids throughout the day while awake because they don't perceive thirst adequately. If a senior sleeps most of the day they might be in a chronically dehydrated state. A variety of favorite drinks should be kept in a covered "sippy" cup within reach. Reminder: older folks might refuse drinking if asked and can forget or ignore the cup of fluid at their bedside. Frequent encouragement and reminders are essential.
- Some general guidelines on daily fluid intake for older adults: As an exercise, take a water-filled 2-liter soda bottle and use it to fill up an 8-ounce cup. What is left in the soda bottle is about 1.75 liters (59 ounces) of fluid since about 30 milliliters (or cc's) equals one ounce of liquid. That 1,750 ml volume that remains in the 2-liter bottle is the average amount of fluid an older adult should take in each day. For seniors below 110 pounds, subtract about 300 milliliters (10 ounces). For older folks weighing above 150 pounds, add about 500 milliliters. Add an additional 500 milliliters daily in those who have fever above 38 degrees Celsius (100.4

Fahrenheit). Assuming a senior is awake 16 hours each day, that means he or she must drink about 3.5 to 4 **ounces** *every hour*!

- Foods with **high water content** can substitute for actual liquids. Approximately 20 percent of our daily water intake comes from food intake. The following list of foods contain more than 80 percent water by weight:
  - Watermelon, honeydew, cantaloupe
  - Grapefruit, pineapple, cherries, grapes, pears, plums, oranges, strawberries and other berries
  - Cucumbers, radishes, tomatoes, green pepper, spinach, eggplant
  - Gelatin desserts, popsicles, soups, ice cream, sherbet, yogurt

Urinary Tract Infections

One tenet of treating older folks is that the elderly have less typical and more unusual presentations of illnesses compared with younger adults. Maybe urinary tract infection (UTI) will be different? Seems fairly straight forward, right? Sadly, that is not the case. UTI in older folks is not a simple diagnosis and is commonly *over-diagnosed* and *over-treated.* Bacteria can live in the urinary tract of old and sick people yet *not* cause active infection. At the other extreme, urinary infections in the elderly can be hidden and subtle, leading to sepsis, dehydration and hospitalization. Some doctors would say it is better to aggressively over-treat a frail senior for *possible* UTI rather than wait two to three days for unreliable test results. The delay might result in hospitalization for dehydration, serious infection or just anxiety and worry by caregiver or family. Christopher J. Crnich, MD PhD, Associate Professor of Medicine, Division of Infectious Diseases, University of Wisconsin School of Medicine and Public Health, might disagree. In personal communications to this author (JC), Dr. Crnich emphasizes that "Antibiotic therapy is not a benign therapeutic intervention." According to Dr. Crnich, 20 percent of all adverse medication reactions in long-term care facilities can be blamed on antibiotics. The risk of suffering from C. Difficile diarrhea, a serious complication of using antibiotics, increases eight-fold following antibiotic exposure and might not show up until several weeks after treatment is completed. Dr. Crnich further stresses that antibiotic resistance is a real concern with overuse of antibiotics. In the adult care home setting, where risks for resistant bacteria and C. Difficile spread are lower than in skilled nursing facilities, Dr. Crnich believes more aggressive and earlier antibiotic use for sudden changes in condition may be more appropriate.

Why is it so difficult to properly diagnose UTI in older folks? Older adults frequently lack typical symptoms like burning with urination, or are unable to convey that information due to memory issues or other communication problems. Another reason: Older folks may already have to urinate frequently, making it hard to assess a change in this sign of UTI. Third, bacteria frequently live in the urinary tract of older folks without causing active infection, the same way some people carry Strep bacteria in their throat without having an acute sore throat. In fact, 20 percent of elderly women living in the community have bacteria harmlessly living in their urinary tract, while up to 50 percent of women in nursing homes will grow bacteria on a urine culture without actively having infection. For elderly men, about 10 percent of those living in the community harbor bacteria in their urinary tract, while up to 40 percent of older men living in nursing homes harbor bacteria in their urine system without an active infection. Urine cultures will grow these bacteria despite recommendations against treating this condition known as "asymptomatic bacteriuria." This ill-advised practice leads to overtreatment based on a urine test that is misleading. This needless treatment with potent antibiotics occurs too commonly in emergency rooms. One recent study published in the *Journal of the American Geriatric Society* found that nearly half of elderly women diagnosed with UTI in an emergency room may have been over-diagnosed. A fourth reason UTI is hard to properly diagnose in older adults is they tend to show vague signs of illness such as weakness, loss of appetite or confusion which can have hundreds of causes other than a urine infection.

Helpful Tips for managing UTI in Older Folks

- If a senior has had similar symptoms before and responded to a short course of antibiotics with return to baseline condition then it is reasonable to treat for that presumed UTI again. Dr. Crnich advocates for this practice as well. If there are clear changes in urine habits or persistent odor change, along with vague new symptoms like loss of appetite or confusion, then a urinary infection is a strong possibility and worth treating.

- Regarding **urine odor** as an indicator of UTI: Treating bad odor is bad practice. Bad odor alone is *not* a reliable indicator of a urinary tract infection. Dr. John Morley, Director of Geriatric Medicine at Saint Louis University School of Medicine, said in a personal communication to this author (JC) that "Over half of smelly urines are *not* urinary tract infections." Dr. Crnich would agree stating, "There is no compelling data that change in odor or clarity (clear versus cloudy) of the urine has any value in predicting the presence of bacteria in the urine." Many factors can alter urine smell and color. Normal urine is pale yellow to yellowish-orange in color. B-vitamins can change the color to bright yellow-green, Carrots or vitamin C can cause orange tinting to urine. Foods such as beets, rhubarb and blackberries might make pee a reddish-pink tint. Regarding odor, asparagus can cause a pungent sulfur smell in urine. Dehydration can cause darker urine with a sharp ammonia smell like floor cleaners due to higher ammonia concentration. Dirty diapers can also become more malodorous as bacteria break down chemical waste into ammonia. Medications can also alter color and odor of urine to various degrees. Commonly used medications can alter urine tint as follows: Senna-reddish; warfarin-orange; promethazine and amitriptyline-greenish; metronidazole and nitrofurantoin (antibiotics)-dark brown or tea color. Blood in urine can turn it reddish to dark brown. Vaginal infections can also contribute to bad urine odor, particular a fishy odor caused by Bacterial Vaginosis. UTI diagnosis is clearly complicated.
- UTI Prevention Strategies: There are a few harmless UTI prevention strategies that are worth using in frail folks prone to urinary infections, none of which have strong scientific evidence they work. Infectious disease expert Dr. Crnich admonishes: "The data on prophylactic antibiotics is clear. It does *not* work and only serves to cultivate (grow) resistant bacteria." Dr. Crnich does advocate trying cranberry tablets (or juice) to help prevent E. Coli urine infections, but he admonishes cranberry may have less benefit for other bacterial causes of UTI. Acidifying the urine can

help prevent urine infections since many of these bacteria flourish in a high-pH (alkaline) environment. How can we get urine to be more acidic? Urine acidification approaches are somewhat murky but the following method may have clearer scientific basis: Vitamin C (ascorbic acid) 1 to 2 grams daily given as a supplement can help lower urine pH. Some studies on urine infections have found a high nitrite concentration in combination with ascorbic acid kills E. Coli bacteria quickly. Green leafy vegetables like spinach contain high levels of nitrates. When nitrates are combined with ascorbic acid in acidic urine, they turn bacterial nitrites into nitrogen oxides which are toxic to bacteria. These nitrogen oxide chemicals have been shown to help kill E. Coli and other bacteria.

The prescription medication **methenamine hippurate** also reduces urine pH and might offer benefit with vitamin C supplements in acidifying urine. Throw in cranberry juice cocktail or tablets, which offer some acidifying benefits and also contain chemicals that directly inhibit bacteria from sticking to the bladder and wreaking havoc. Now you have a recipe for naturally preventing UTI without excessive antibiotic use! The goal is to reduce urine pH below 5.0 to 6.0. I recommend purchasing an inexpensive pack of **urine pH test strips** to check urine pH periodically by collecting urine in a clean tray, or placing a test strip under the urine stream. Testing urine pH is a simple way to track if the measures discussed above are sufficient and effective in acidifying the urine to help reduce recurring urinary tract infections. Acetic acid (white vinegar) diluted to a 1:20 ratio with water to irrigate the bladder through a urinary catheter may also be an effective approach whereby home health nurses can acidify urine. If ordered by a doctor, this procedure helps to reduce bacteria and sediment in urine.

"Goodbye-UTI" Recipe:

Cranberry:

Three to 4 ounces cranberry juice *cocktail* twice or three times daily or

One ounce 100 percent cranberry juice once or twice daily or

One gram of *concentrated* cranberry extract twice daily or

One to 3 cranberry *capsules* daily (36 milligrams cranberry proanthocyanidin) or

Cranberry liquid blend 60 milliliters daily

Vitamin C (ascorbic acid):

1000 milligrams once or twice daily to help acidify urine

Methenamine Hippurate Tablets:

One gram once or twice daily to acidify urine (hippuric acid). This is available only by prescription in the United States. Large tablets can be split or crushed. Enteric coated tablets should not be crushed. Drink a full glass of water to wash this pill down. It can cause stomach upset. Avoid this medication in those with significant kidney or liver damage.

Prune Juice:

Prune juice is moderately acidic with an average pH of 4.0. This might help acidify urine in theory as no scientific studies have been done to show benefit. The other advantage: less constipation. Drink 2 ounces prune juice once or twice daily.

Leafy Green Vegetables:

No specific study exists to prove benefit or quantify a dose but the theory is higher urinary nitrate levels get converted into nitrogen oxides in acidic urine. These nitrogen oxides are highly toxic to bacteria. Spinach and kale are fine options. Be cautious if taking warfarin blood thinners!

Avoid Citrus:

Lemon, lime, oranges, grapefruit are all acidic but paradoxically turn the urine more alkaline, undoing the above recipe goals. These citrus juices, however, can help to reduce formation of most types of kidney stones.

Beware:

Beware of acid reflux or stomach upset with this recipe. Beware of eating excess greens if taking the blood thinner, warfarin. Beware that most kidney stones are more likely to form in acid urine.

A WORD ON BLADDER CATHETERS

Between 20 and 50 percent of bladder catheters are inserted unnecessarily and without clear rationale, as mentioned in the Hospitalization Risks chapter. Potential serious complications of catheters include resistant urine infections and sepsis. These tubes can reduce quality of life as well. Some key tips for caregivers:

▶ Always advocate for a healthcare provider to discontinue a catheter, if possible. Safer alternatives should be considered when a catheter is necessary such as intermittent (in and out) catheterization, condom catheters placed over the penis, or a surgically placed suprapubic catheter. Adult briefs are surely safer than an indwelling urine catheter.

▶ Minimize tinkering with the closed-bag collection system to avoid bacterial contamination.

▶ For long term use, the International Continence Society recommends silicone and hydrogel catheters.

▶ Bladder catheters are typically ***not*** recommended for the inconvenience of incontinence.

▶ All people with indwelling catheters have colonies of bacteria growing along the inner lining of these tubes within a few days. Sending a urine culture based upon urine appearance only is wasteful and could lead to unnecessary intravenous antibiotic treatment. The test will always return a "positive" growth of bacteria. That is why doctors should only diagnose UTI in folks with catheters when they are suddenly sick. Typical signs may include fever, back pain, abdominal pain, bladder spasms with urine leakage, loss of appetite or vomiting, sudden lethargy or sleeping much more. The urine test alone is meaningless if that person feels fine or the same as usual. Pus from serious infection in the urine can make urine appear like milk in the tubing. This is also concerning and needs immediate action. Pockets of sediment or "crud" between clearer-looking urine is common and needs action to prevent tube clogging, but does not automatically mean there is an infection.

▶ Diabetics and older folks are more prone to have bacteria living in their urinary system without causing active infection.

▶ When a senior returns from the hospital with a diagnosis of UTI and is to continue antibiotics, Dr. Crnich advises that providers consider reducing the dose and perhaps the duration of treatment if there is clear improvement in their condition. This can prevent side effects or too-high dosing in a frail senior who might even have been over-diagnosed by the emergency room.

Cough in Older Adults

Older folks can suffer from pneumonia and *not* have a cough or fever. When an older adult does have a persistent cough lasting more than three weeks, it is usually caused by the same three culprits, or a combination of these, as in younger adults: postnasal drip from a cold or allergies or sinus infection, asthma and/or acid reflux. What is most important for caregivers to identify is any red flag symptoms that accompany that cough. Red flag symptoms include shortness of breath symptoms (see also, Shortness of Breath chapter), fever, loss of appetite, weight loss, unusual weakness or sleepiness, unusual confusion or loss of a functional ability. These suggest the cough is more serious. Other concerns would include increasing ankle swelling since heart failure can cause a cough. In addition, blood in the phlegm more than once can be a sign of tuberculosis or lung cancer. Aspiration is also more likely in older folks, especially if they cough a lot during meals or while drinking. Since the cough reflex is crucial in preventing aspiration (lung inhalation of food), it is best *not* to suppress a cough with cough suppressants. Treating the underlying causes of a persistent cough is a wiser strategy. Sedating drugs also increase susceptibility to aspiration. Deep breathing exercises daily, cupping and clapping the back, and use of incentive spirometers (rising ball when sucking in air) to expand the lungs can be helpful.

Click on the website for more caregiver advice on managing common problems in older folks:

www.EmergencyRoomSurvivalBookForOlderAdults.com

V. SHORTNESS OF BREATH: IS IT SERIOUS?

As breathing goes, aging is not kind to us. So many body changes spanning years of wear and tear transform breathing from automatic to effortful. There is even a failure in the aging body's ability to recognize breathing compromise. The consequence is that older folks may delay seeking help when serious breathing trouble strikes.

Loss of muscle mass as we gray weakens between-rib and diaphragm muscles that play a key role in easy breathing. Arthritic changes, hunched back, wear-and-tear calcium deposits, and scarred body tissue all contribute to chest rigidity. This makes breathing a chore, like blowing up a balloon that has been coated with paper mâché. Other factors that magnify respiratory compromise include less efficient contaminant-clearing cilia that line the interior of breathing passages, reduced cough effectiveness, and greater risk of lung aspiration from aging brain diseases.

When breathing difficulty appears where do doctors look first? The heart and lungs. The brain is an occasional culprit, usually in the form of anxiety.

The sensation of shortness of breath or air hunger strikes a chord of fear and panic even in the most stoic among us. Some common causes for breathing difficulty include heart failure, asthma, emphysema, pneumonia, allergic reaction, anxiety and hyperventilation. Sometimes air hunger is ongoing and chronic, at other times breathing trouble is sudden, severe and requires immediate action to prevent crisis. In either case, there is increased effort and work to breathe. Fortunately, several signs exist to suggest breathing trouble is more likely to be serious or imminently life-threatening.

- **General Appearance**: Those who suffer from breathing compromise of any cause might show any of the following body responses to air hunger:
  - * Eyes prominent and almost bulging
  - * Sitting or standing up in a "tripod" position – leaning forward with hands or arms resting on knees or another surface, usually working hard to suck in air

  * Labored breathing with accessory neck and chest muscles contracting frantically to help suck more air into the lungs
  * Confusion, restlessness, anxiety, severe sweating
  * At the other extreme, inability to wake up or lethargic when breathing failure and death loom near

- **Speech**: Choppy speech – saying few words then gasping for air, or minimal speaking suggests trouble is brewing. If the person is having a full conversation with you then there is time to try simple treatments or to get an urgent medical evaluation.
- **Color**: Pallor or paleness can be a sign of low levels of red blood cells (anemia), insufficient blood circulation, or not enough oxygen in red blood cells to turn blood bright red. Cyanosis is a bluish-purple tinge to nail beds of fingers or lips when breathing is severely compromised. Think purple lips when someone stays too long in an outdoor pool.
- **Other Key Symptoms, signs and Complaints**: Other worrisome symptoms or signs include chest discomfort, feeling faint, ankle swelling in both legs, severe fatigue with daily activities, coughing and increased phlegm, fever, and sudden inability to eat or persistent nausea. Weight gain of more than two to three pounds can also be a reliable sign of fluid retention from heart failure, especially if breathing worsens as weight increases.
- **Timing of Illness:** Breathing trouble that gradually worsens over one to three days is not as worrisome as sudden, severe breathing compromise within minutes to hours. Sudden, rapid and severe shortness of breath usually justifies calling 911 for a trip to the emergency room. Gradual progression allows time to catch the problem earlier, use established treatments (like nebulizer treatment or diuretics), and to get a prompt medical evaluation.
- **Mental Status:** Older folks who become oxygen-starved commonly become increasingly restless, agitated, confused, disoriented or even sleepy and lethargic.

Normal vs. Abnormal Breathing Patterns: Normal breathing is quiet, effortless and easy. A normal range for breathing rate is about 12 to 18 breaths per minute in adults. Those who live in a long term care setting can average as much as 16 to 25 breaths per minute at their baseline. Above 20 breaths per minute in healthier adults and above 25 breaths per minute in frail adults is definitely considered abnormal if it is a new finding. Count the number of breaths for 30 seconds then multiply by a factor of two to calculate respiratory rate. Signs of labored or hard-work breathing include grunting, deeper and more rapid breathing, widening (flaring) of nostrils during inspiration, pursed lip breathing, and prominence or bulging effect of the eyes. A person with breathing compromise usually will display open-mouth breathing as well. At the other extreme, breathing failure can lead to shallow, infrequent breaths with each breath coming after a few second pause. This signifies the end of the line if machine-based breathing support does not come quickly.

- **Chest Sounds**: Musical whistling, crackling or bubbling sounds comprise the symphonic medley that might be playing inside the chest from active heart and lung disease. Use a stethoscope or your ear upon the back or chest to tune in.
- **Position**: Cannot lie flat, Sitting in "tripod position" leaning forward with elbows resting on legs or straightened arms grasping the bed to support upper body – like a camera tripod.
- **Muscle Retractions**: Twitching contractions of the muscles between ribs can be visible to the eye when there is trouble in breathing paradise. Muscles above the collar bone into the neck also assist with breathing and they will be twitching and contracting vigorously to help suck in more air.
- **Rapid Breathing Rate**: Increased rate of this vital sign is a red flag that something is not right – from anxiety or fever to new medical crises, or simply worsening of a chronic disease such as heart failure or emphysema. Count the number of breaths for 30 seconds then multiply by a factor of two to calculate respiratory rate. Know the baseline breathing rate range of frail folks so any change to a persistently higher respiratory rate will be an early clue trouble is brewing.
- **Rapid Heart Rate**: When body cells are oxygen starved, the heart will kick it into high gear and pump harder and faster to

get nutrients to vital organs. A clear increase in heart rate above baseline values can also serve as a valuable *early* clue something is amiss – from fever to anemia to anxiety to heart or lung ailments. A prompt medical evaluation is best to find and treat the cause.

- **Abdominal Muscle Paradox**: During normal breathing the lower rib cage expands out and upwards in synch with abdominal muscles bulging outward. During inspiration, if the abdominal wall muscles draw inward (rather than normal outward ballooning) while the rib cage expands outward, this can be a clear sign of respiratory compromise.
- **At Rest Versus Exertional Breathing Trouble**: Chronic heart and lung problems in older folks frequently cause gradual worsening of breathing or easy fatigue with basic daily activities. This is the early window of time to get medical evaluation and treatment before hospitalization becomes necessary. That point when an ER visit is needed often reveals itself with significant or worse air hunger even while the person is at complete *rest*. The goal is to prevent breathing deterioration from getting to this point.

Simple Steps to Manage Shortness of Breath

1. Encourage slow deep breaths in through the nose, count to five, then out through the mouth. Encouragement to maximize the mechanics of breathing while keeping an eye on the person and offering reassurance can go a long way until medical help arrives.
2. Check vital signs including blood pressure, heart rate, breathing rate. Any significant change from baseline values for that person? Any indication of fever? Any weight gain if a weight check on a scale is possible?
3. Listen to the front and back of the person's chest for wheezing or gurgling sounds using a decent quality stethoscope or by placing your ear on the back and chest. Abnormal sounds can give clues to the underlying cause for air hunger.
4. Are there any simple treatments that can be given to that person that they get regularly or have gotten in the past to help alleviate

air hunger? For instance, a nebulizer treatment (emphysema or asthma) or extra diuretic pills (heart failure) or antibiotic if lung infection is suspected.

5. If oxygen is available through a concentrator or portable tank then hook it up and watch for improvements such as pinker skin color; slower heart rate; and easier, less rapid breathing.
6. Keep handy a finger oxygen saturation gadget (pulse oximeter) to monitor blood oxygen levels. Above 90 percent is usually sufficient but if someone drops to 90 from a usual 99 percent it may signal serious trouble. Decent quality finger pulse oximeter gadgets can be purchased online for less than 50 dollars.
7. If the person is having difficulty coughing up mucus then gently cupping and clapping your curved palm up and down their back may loosen up thick phlegm. This can make it easier to cough up mucus and clear the breathing passages. Also encourage drinking more fluids to thin out the secretions and slower, deeper breaths.

VI. TIPS TO MANAGE FEVER

Humanity has but three great enemies: fever, famine and war. Of these, by far the greatest, by far the most terrible, is fever.

Sir William Osler, 19th Century Physician

On a cold and snowy Saturday evening Henry felt under the weather so he went to bed early. During the night he awoke soaked in a sweat and chilly on drenched sheets. The 66-year-old man had a hard time getting a full, deep breath and felt feverish. "I feel like death warmed over," he told his wife with a chuckle.

"Should I call the doctor?" his wife asked.

"No, they'll just tell me to take an aspirin and drink a glass of water," Henry joked. So he took an aspirin, washed it down with water and went back to bed.

The following morning Henry felt like a truckload of bricks rested on his body. He could barely get out of bed. His wife took his temperature: 103 degrees!

Henry's wife was near panic. A whirlwind of thoughts swirled inside her head. Should she drive her husband to the emergency room? Call 911? Call their family doctor? Try a nurse help line? Or wait another day or two giving him soups and fever-lowering pills?

What should Henry and his wife do?

Fever in Adults

Fever has been recognized as the hallmark of illness since the time of Hippocrates. So important is fever as a measure of illness, it is included as one of the four original "Vital Signs" which includes pulse, blood pressure, and breathing rate. These vitals are taken at every clinic visit and every ER encounter. When hospitalized, vitals are measured every few hours during the entire hospitalization, much to the chagrin of sleep-deprived patients.

What temperature defines a fever? Normal temperature in adults varies throughout the day between 98°F to as high as 100°F (36. 8 -37.8°C). Body temperature trends lower in the early morning and higher at about dinnertime. Most experts consider a temperature above 100.3°F (38°C) to be a fever in healthier adults. High fevers are those above 102.5°F up to 103.9°F (39.2 -39.9°C). Very high fevers are those above 104°F (40°C). Why is this important? High fevers in older adults need prompt medical evaluation. And very high fevers need immediate medical evaluation and treatment, either from an urgent care facility or emergency room.

Fever in Older Folks

The rules change when older adults who suffer from several chronic illnesses spike a fever or appear ill. Up to one-third of elderly patients who have an infection do not ever mount a fever response. This is especially true for frail elderly. What exactly is a frail older adult? You would likely identify one if you saw a frail person. Frailty is somewhat controversial but is broadly defined as a body no longer able to adjust to outside stresses – a breakdown in body balance or homeostasis. Key apparent features of frailty include weight loss, weakness, feeling fatigued most of the day, and slow walking speed. If frail elders spike a fever, take it seriously since they often do not so ominous causes may be brewing.

Fever in older adults with chronic illnesses and in frail folks is defined as temperature above 99°F or 37.2°C. Another measure that might be more accurate is a *rise* in temperature of 1.5 degrees above that individual's *baseline* body temperature. This must be measured using a consistent procedure with the same thermometer type and similar time of day for baseline values.

Fever in older adults can also be caused by diseases that are not infections such as cancers or autoimmune diseases like Lupus or Rheumatoid Arthritis.

Factors Indicating Fever Might be More Serious

▶ Presence of frailty

▶ Confusion or agitation

▶ Feeling very weak or drowsy, hard to arouse

▶ Temperature above 101°F in older folks

▶ Loss of appetite

▶ Loss of functional ability like standing or walking

▶ Falling

▶ Fever accompanied by abdominal pain, trouble breathing or having a new cough, experiencing diarrhea or vomiting also add significantly to concern about a fever.

▶ Those who have diabetes, cancer, or advanced kidney disease may have reduced immunity, making fever a sign of potentially serious infections

▶ Medications that suppress immunity include prednisone, methotrexate, cyclosporin and many newer specialized drugs, all of which can predispose these people to serious infections

▶ Living in a nursing home or assisted living facility, many of whom are frail

Factors Indicating Fever is Less Likely to be Serious

▶ Normal behavior

- Normal appetite
- No loss of functional abilities
- Able to participate in usual daily activities of living

Tips to Manage Fever in Older Adults

1. Keep a thermometer handy and the battery charged. See Red Flags chapter for an additional section on fever and thermometer accuracy concerns.
2. Keep the room comfortably cool, but not too cold to cause shivering and chilly discomfort. Older folks like to dress in several layers of clothing, even during the summer. When a senior has possible fever, it is important to keep them in only one layer of light cotton clothing so they are able to evaporate sweat, allowing the body to cool down. Avoid the piles of wool blankets and replace them with one sheet or thin covering.
3. Push plenty of fluids, including soups, juices, coffee, teas, sports drinks, milk or water.
4. Lukewarm baths may ease the discomfort. But do not bathe or shower in cold water since it will prevent heat evaporation and natural cooling inside the body.
5. Take it easy, no strenuous exercise or outdoor activity.
6. Do not sponge down with rubbing alcohol since this can be toxic.
7. Fever causes muscle breakdown and fluid loss – two body stresses older folks cannot afford. High temperature also increases work demands of the heart and lungs which might tip a delicate balance in those with diseases of these vital organs. It is advisable to reduce the fever despite the theory that higher body temperature fights off infection-causing bacteria or viruses. Acetaminophen 500 mg is the safest first line medication treatment (after cool room and light clothing). Ibuprofen 200 to 400 mg or naproxen 220 mg are also off-the-shelf fever-reducing medications that can be used. Ibuprofen and naproxen must be used more judiciously since they can cause stomach ulcers, worsening heart failure and increase high blood pressure in susceptible people. General comfort and

relief from muscle aches, shivers and lassitude are also a reasonable motivation to quash a spiking fever.

As for Henry and his fever, since he was in overall good health, he did not have to rush to an emergency room. He called his doctor but could not get in for another three days. There was no urgent care center nearby that Henry had faith in. Henry's wife wisely would not wait so long so they were evaluated in their community hospital emergency room. That fever spike of 103°F was a key clue that even healthy Henry needed prompt evaluation and treatment. Final ER diagnosis: pneumonia. It took Henry two weeks to recover his usual energy and motivation to do yard work.

SECTION VI. APPENDIX A

PLANNING AHEAD FOR EMERGENCIES

Step 1: Locate a quality community hospital and university or teaching hospital in your area. Get recommendations from friends, doctors, nurses in your area. Search the website of those hospitals and emergency rooms. Do they offer expertise relevant to your medical history such as a chest pain unit in the emergency department and 24-7 emergency heart procedure availability to treat heart attacks? Is the teaching hospital a level 1 trauma center for serious injuries or burns? Does the hospital offer specialized neurologic disease expertise for dementia or Parkinson's disease, for instance? A trusted local community hospital can be valuable for common variety illness such as a kidney stone or asthma attack. Waits will likely be shorter and you are less likely to get treatment from a student or doctor-in-training.

Step 2: Map out quick routes to your hospitals of choice. Also write down the phone number for a local ambulance or fire department service if your town offers volunteer emergency transport.

Step 3: Read published reviews and rankings of the care and procedures offered by those hospitals. US News, Medicare rankings, State Health Department rankings for heart procedures, for instance. Online searches can locate this information with a little effort.

Step 4: Find a specialist you trust in your area for a serious illness such as a cardiologist for heart disease. Be sure to get the on-call page system information for emergency contact.

Step 5: Find a trusted urgent care clinic in your neighborhood based upon recommendations from friends, relatives, nurses or doctors. This can be a useful resource to avoid the hospital ER for less serious ailments or injuries.

Step 6: Develop a good relationship with a primary care doctor who will see you within 24 hours when you suffer unexpected illness. Your PCP should be a valuable asset for guiding you with tough care decisions and getting you needed help on short notice.

Step 7: Enter your key "crisis information" onto the inner covers of BoomER book so you have this information at your fingertips if medical crisis strikes.

Step 8: Keep an updated list of all prescription and off-the-shelf medications, supplements and herbal remedies you take.

Step 9: I recommend that anybody over age 45 years get a baseline electrocardiogram, shrink it down to wallet size and have it laminated. This will prove vital for doctors to use as comparison if you ever develop a suspected heart problem.

Step 10: Consider getting a Medic Alert Bracelet as warning about any serious medical conditions or allergies you suffer from.

Step 11: If you have decided against aggressive care interventions like chest compressions or breathing tube and machine, prepare an orange (or other color) Do Not Resuscitate (DNR) form or POLST form and keep it on your refrigerator. Some states offer DNR bracelets for those who wish to avoid extraordinary or aggressive treatments when in the final phase of life. Notify local ambulance crews and emergency rooms of your wishes and send a copy of your POLST or DNR medical order for limited care to these places (See also, Last Wishes chapter).

Step 12: An ounce of prevention is worth a pound of treatment. Note all heart attack and stroke risk factors mentioned in this book that apply to you. Begin lifestyle modifications to improve your future heart attack and stroke risk profile. Reduction in disease risk factors for high blood pressure, diabetes, heart disease and stroke can also help minimize your risks for dementia, leg artery disease (peripheral arterial disease), and erectile dysfunction.

Step 13: Aggressively discuss with your doctor reducing medication burden once you pass three or four medications on your list. Recall that chances for adverse reactions to medications approaches 100 percent once you reach seven or more medications! There is clearly a point at which more and more drugs do more harm than good, especially in those who are frail or have many chronic illnesses. Long med lists can surely lead to avoidable ER visits and hospital admissions.

SECTION VII. APPENDIX B
CONSIDER ALTERNATIVES TO EMERGENCY ROOM CARE

When someone falls ill the mind starts racing. What is the most likely ailment that I have? Maybe I should try an off-the-shelf remedy or just take a nap? Should I rush to the emergency room? Which one? Do I need an ambulance? Is this problem life threatening? Am I going to die? If my symptoms are not too bad, what other options do I have if I am to avoid emergency room chaos? Can I even afford the costly medical bills that will be pouring in?

Some simple answers and a wise strategy follow below. First, plan ahead (see also, Appendix A). Do not give these questions your first thought when you have already fallen ill. Develop your strategy today. A proactive plan is particularly important for older adults who have several chronic ailments and who are at greater risk for suffering from serious disease when sudden symptoms strike.

First Line of Defense: Prevent Problems when Possible

Not to beat a dead horse, so to speak, but this point cannot be overemphasized. Strive to shrink your medication list to reduce inevitable side effects. Become a drug skeptic, not a medication magnet. Drug doses and uses are dynamic; treatment needs change over time with body changes and new health situations. Medication necessity and dose should be reassessed every few months. Falls are also a major cause for injury and death in older folks. Clear out walking paths in your home and wear non-slip shoes to avoid trips and falls. Use a cane or walker or other assist device if needed. Resist the temptation to climb onto a stool or ladder to change a light bulb: that stool might as well be Mount Everest. It may not end well. Exercise to maintain muscle strength since functional decline is a major contributor to emergency room use, loss of independence and need for nursing home care. Install bathroom safety devices such as a grab bars, shower chair, non-slip mat, and raised toilet seat. Cushion sharp furniture edges to limit fall injuries. Eat several smaller meals throughout day. Avoid living alone, if possible, especially if getting around the house is becoming a chore.

Second Line of Defense: Find a Quality Primary Care or House-Call Doctor

Find a healthcare provider who is available to evaluate and treat you for urgencies without immediately shipping you off to an emergency room. Get a doctor or other healthcare provider who asks you what your wishes and goals for care are; one who is interested in your life story and who you are as a person; one who aims to *limit* tests, drugs and treatments whenever possible; one who understands the dangers of hospitalization and who strives to keep you safe from emergency room chaos and hospital hazards, whenever possible.

Third Line of Defense: Trusted Community Urgent Care Facility

Do friends and neighbors recommend a local facility based upon positive experiences they have had? Search for nearby urgent care or walk-in practices online or spot one as you drive through the neighborhood. Determine if they have had many online complaints or a pattern of negative reviews. One or two negative comments should not be a deciding factor since nobody pleases all the people all of the time. Is it staffed by well-trained doctors? Or less-trained, but competent, professionals such as a nurse practitioner or physician assistant? Do providers have emergency care experience? Are doctors and NPs board certified? Are they experienced in caring for the elderly? Next, take a trip to the chosen facility to check out how chaotic or efficient the place is. Speak with front-desk staff and find out if you can ask a nurse or doctor some questions that come to mind.

Fourth Line of Defense: Freestanding Emergency Rooms

These somewhat controversial care facilities are equipped to treat more serious illnesses. Some people have described them as ritzy urgent care facilities with triple the expense to patients. Freestanding emergency rooms are not attached to hospitals. They have sprung up in about 40 states, but remain concentrated in states such as Florida, Texas, Georgia and Colorado. These pseudo-emergency rooms might initiate treatment for serious problems like a heart attack, but will have to transfer seriously ill folks by ambulance to the nearest hospital. This extra step ultimately delays time-dependent treatment. Even if the well-trained ER doctor staffed at a freestanding facility did administer clot-dissolving treatment for a heart attack, for example, that facility does not often perform these treatments compared to volume in a hospital-based emergency room. Would you prefer receiving a risky treatment from those who do that procedure or treatment every day, or from those who have far less experience? In addition, specialists are likely to be less available to see you while you are at a freestanding ER.

Some advantages to this option do exist: Nicer, quieter and generally more pleasant environment; shorter waits for care; possible close proximity to home; more likely to be staffed by a board-certified and experienced emergency care physician compared to an urgent care or walk-in clinic. Depending upon whether the freestanding ER accepts full payment from your insurer and if your illness is unlikely to be life-threatening, these better-equipped care facilities can be a quieter alternative for getting quality emergency care. Common variety ailments and injuries such as dehydration from a stomach virus, asthma attack, kidney stone, migraine headache, and slip and fall are all appropriate for this care venue. Urgent care might be equipped to manage these illnesses as well but it depends largely on the training and experience of the health professional working that shift.

SECTION VIII. APPENDIX C

PERSON IN BLUE SCRUBS OR WHITE COAT – KNOW WHO IS TREATING YOU IN THE EMERGENCY ROOM

In an emergency, the type of doctor who takes care of you is important and may make the difference between life and death. You want the best-trained and most experienced physician for complex and life-threatening illness.

Imagine arriving in an ER after being bitten by a rattlesnake. Your throbbing leg resembles an elephant leg, and your body throbs from pain. But the treating doctor only works two shifts per month to earn extra money to supplement income in addition to his health insurance desk job. He is not board certified in Emergency Medicine and has surely never seen a rattlesnake bite, or for that matter, a rattlesnake. The "moonlighting" doctor searches rattlesnake bites on the internet and stumbles upon an unreliable website. Without having had formal training in snakebite management, the doctor implements the questionable advice found on that website: "Treatment should consist of pain medication and antihistamines," the unreliable site recommends. The snakebite victim is then left in the crowded corridor – only to be found dead several hours later.

So who are the people who could be treating you in the emergency room?

Larger teaching hospital (university) emergency rooms may have many people involved in your care. Your head may be spinning, in fact, from the attention overdose. Smaller community hospital ERs usually have only one ER physician, and a handful of nurses. Here is a summary of personnel types that can be involved in treating you during your emergency room visit:

Emergency Medicine Board-Certified Physicians

This is this highest level of physicians staffing ERs in the US. The good news is that most doctors working in ERs are board certified in Emergency Medicine. The vast majority of these physicians have completed a rigorous four-year formal Emergency Medicine residency training program at a university hospital. A smaller percentage of full-time ER physicians are trained in other specialties such as Internal Medicine, Family Practice or General Surgery but have years of emergency room care experience.

What's special about physicians who are board certified in Emergency medicine? Here are a few of the abilities they have:

1. Within minutes, determine who is really critically sick of injured. You might think it would be obvious, but some people near death may appear okay to the untrained eye.
2. Provide lifesaving interventions like placing special intravenous fluid lines into someone who is hemorrhaging.
3. Pass a breathing tube into a person's windpipe (intubation). This can save a life if the patient has stopped breathing.
4. Perform CPR and advanced support resuscitation on folks rushed to the emergency room in critical condition.
5. Rapidly identify and treat heart attacks or strokes, two time-dependent acute illnesses.
6. Treat major injuries from auto crashes.
7. Decide who needs admission to the hospital for further care.
8. Diagnose and set dislocated or broken bones.
9. Provide relief from severe pain.
10. Treat serious infections, like meningitis, pneumonia and sepsis.
11. Take care of critically ill or injured children.
12. Perform procedures such as repairing lacerations (cuts), draining

abscesses, placing chest tubes for a collapsed lung, and lumbar punctures to diagnose possible meningitis.

13. Deliver babies.
14. Determine the type of specialist needed for advanced care.
15. Treat snakebites, spider bites, and allergic reactions to bees.
16. Treat overdoses and poisonings from numerous drugs or toxins.
17. Determine if serious problems are the cause for your abdominal pain.
18. Treat heatstroke and cold exposure

Moonlighters

Some non-ER physicians seek weekend or evening jobs to gain extra income. This group is referred to by some of their colleagues as "Weekend Warriors." The term "moonlighter" means a physician who is dedicated full time to *another* specialty, and is hired because the ER needs night-time or weekend shifts filled. You should worry about this group because most do not have the proper training experience to handle certain serious emergencies. They may have taken a few hours of advanced training such as advanced cardiac life support (ACLS), advanced Trauma Life support (ATLS), or Advanced Pediatric life support. These "merit badge" courses do not substitute for rigorous training or experience.

Physicians in Training

If you get care at a teaching hospital you may well get initial care from a physician-in-training. This can include medical students, interns (first-year doctor), or residents in a variety of specialties, such as family practice, internal medicine, surgery, anesthesiology and others. If the hospital has an emergency medicine training program, an ER resident could also see you. Teaching hospitals theoretically require all cases be discussed with an experienced attending physician but this rarely happens during busy times. And these emergency departments are almost always busy.

Nurses

Nurses are an integral and valuable part of emergency rooms, No nurses, no ERs. A nurse's role in providing care has expanded over the years. As noted in other chapters nurse responsibility also includes sorting of initial illness severity (triage). Once you are in the emergency room the nurses are responsible for periodic assessments of signed-in patients to determine if their condition changes. They should notify the doctor if a patient deteriorates. They are the ones who will also dispense your medications including pain medications. They will comfort you during times of distress (e.g. vomiting, severe pain, scary procedures). They can be your best friends in the ER, and have great insights into many common patient questions. Nurses must also endure a great deal of stress in emergency rooms so please be courteous to them, even when you must work hard to get needed attention. Nurses are on your side, so stay on theirs.

Mid-level Healthcare Providers

Mid-level providers generally fall into two categories: nurse practitioners (NPs) or physician assistants (PAs). Although training and license requirements differ, they are both considered physician extenders and can offer experience in treating "bread and butter" ailments they see often in the ER. Each of the fifty states has laws which govern their practice, and how much independence they have from physicians. Mid-level practitioners are generally assigned less complex and severe cases. They take histories, perform physical examinations, order lab tests and imaging studies, and initiate treatment with medications. They may sew up the cut on your arm, or splint your ankle sprain. In some ERs they discuss your case with the attending physician before you are released. In others, their charts may be reviewed after the fact. Sometimes the mid-levels are assigned cases which appear simple, but turn out to be serious. If the mid-level does not recognize their limits, errors can be made. This same principle, however, applies to doctors as well.

ER Technicians

The ER technician may smile and talk with you more than other staff in the ER. In distant years they were also referred to as "orderlies." Increased job training and complexity have earned them a new title and greater respect for this valuable emergency department team member. They do everything asked of them by nurses and physicians, some of which might include getting needed equipment in a hurry, performing an electrocardiogram, transporting patients for important tests, assisting patients with toileting or other comfort needs, and much more.

Pharmacists

More hospitals are hiring pharmacists to help oversee medication use in emergency rooms and increasing their involvement in patient care. Pharmacists spend several years in school after college and have a "Doctor of Pharmacy" degree. If present in the ER and involved in your care they should introduce themselves. They may ask you questions about medications you have taken, and explain more complex drugs given to you in that high-stakes setting.

Emergency Room Volunteers

Volunteers in the emergency department are generally young students or older retirees with an interest in helping others. Some plan to get advanced training and then formally enter the medical field. "Candy Striper," may come to mind when thinking about the stereotypical hospital volunteer. During World War II, these Candy Stripers were young women who volunteered to give support to needy hospitals. Now volunteers may be comprised of high school or college students, pre-med students, pre-nursing students, and retirees with time to spare and motivation to give back to the community. These volunteers generally perform simple tasks when asked by the nursing staff. If you ask a question, they will usually defer to the nurse or doctor providing care for you.

ER Research Techs

University emergency rooms are always doing research to improve care. You might encounter a young person with a clipboard who will ask you if you are willing to participate in a study. The study may involve answering a set of questions or consenting to receive a new medication. Give careful thought before accepting untested treatments or drugs.

A Few Patient Tips:

1. Ask each person involved in your care to identify him or herself. They should explain their role in your care and have an identification badge to confirm their status.
2. If you are in a teaching hospital, ask to see the attending physician at some point in your care. Be sure to ask that senior-most doctor probing questions. The attending physician in charge is your go-to person if your condition is not improving or if you have concerns about the experience of the provider caring for you, the tests being ordered, or the attention you are not receiving.
3. If you receive care from a mid-level provider and are unsatisfied, ask to speak to the ER physician in charge for another opinion and a "double-check" evaluation. If the emergency department doctor in charge does not adequately address your concerns then you can request an appropriate specialist's opinion.
4. How can you tell if your doctor is Board Certified in Emergency Medicine? Simply ask the doctor. For providers with other training fields or levels, use your instinct and judgment as to whether you trust they are on the right track and are providing thorough, common sense, wise and compassionate care.

SECTION IX. APPENDIX D

BEWARE HOSPITAL DISCHARGE DANGERS

BE AWARE OF these emergency room or hospital discharge pitfalls that could have disheartening or deadly consequences. When you are being positioned on the emergency room or hospital launching pad, and the doctor is preparing to send you home, never leave that ER (or hospital) unless you are feeling much improved, fully understand your condition and treatment, and know who to call for timely outside follow up care. Following are a few ER discharge dangers to steer clear of:

- **Half-treatment:** This might be called "incompletely stabilized" and usually occurs during the most chaotic of times. For example, an asthmatic is given a nebulizer treatment to help with easier breathing. The doctor sees some improvement so immediately insists on quick discharge with additional treatment at home. If you feel uneasy and are not significantly improved and monitored for a while even after improvement, you are at risk for a dangerous discharge.

Solution: Don't leave the ER treatment area until you feel much improved. If not much better, tell the doctor or nurse you are still too ill to go home and require additional monitoring, support and medical care.

- **Sending you home when you require hospital admission:** Sometimes patients are sent home when they are at risk for deterioration or complications. For instance, a doctor tells you that you have pneumonia, but thinks you can be treated at home. He cites your score of 65 points on the pneumonia "PORT admission scale" and this means you qualify for care at home since above 70 points justifies admission. This might be great news for frail folks who ideally should stay away from the hospital, but if you feel too sick to manage at home or lack sufficient support resources, then mention your concerns before you become a discharge danger victim.

Solution: Tell the doctor you are too sick to go home. If you get nowhere, insist on a second opinion or have your family doctor explain your situation if your pleas fall on deaf ears. Perhaps request that a specialist come see you, if necessary.

- **Getting insufficient discharge instructions:** Most ERs in the United States have adapted electronic medical records. Discharge instructions are usually printed from a computer program, based on your discharge diagnosis. In some cases patients are sent home with discharge instructions so long and confusing that they become essentially worthless. The authors have seen discharge instructions over a dozen pages long containing much textbook or theoretical information rather than three or four salient points that individual needs to know. There was once a time when the physician or nurse would write in their own handwriting a few crucial instructions and warnings that were practical and could be absorbed. Sadly, the long discharge dissertations printed for patients do little to inform the primary care doctor about what happened during the ER visit. A prompt follow up visit with the primary care doctor will lose some value when records must still be requested from the hospital. A brief summary of diagnoses, key test results, treatments given and any complications or concerns would be short and most helpful. Needless to say, any written info must be legible. Do not let staff rush you out before you can comfortably read all paperwork and instructions.

Solution: If you do not understand the three or four points you most need to know when you are discharged, ask the doctor or nurse to slowly explain them and jot down the crucial points in large, legible handwriting. Make your own notes in the margins of the discharge summary. Decline signing your ER exit papers until you fully understand what your likely diagnosis is, what you should do to continue to improve (assuming you have improved already), and with whom you must get follow up care and in how long.

- **Do not get referred to a nonexistent primary care physician (PCP):** Emergency rooms try to reduce their liability by telling patients to follow up with their physician or one whom they recommend and scribble illegibly on discharge paperwork. The dilemma: many patients do not have a family doctor. For those folks who do, it might take weeks to be seen in follow up. There are recent reports in parts of the United States that finding a new primary care doctor can take up to one year and follow ups can be pushed back three months! Suppose you suffer from a brutal headache, for instance. The ER physician orders a brain CT scan and tells you all is okay – no brain tumor or bleeding in the brain. You are quickly sent home but your head pain returns by the time potent pain medication given to you runs out. Will you now have to suffer for weeks until your follow up appointment? Will you have to return to the emergency room if the migraine peaks again?

Solution: Tell the ER doctor that you do not have immediate follow-up and that you require a prescription for a few weeks of effective, safe and affordable medication to treat symptoms. If you lack a PCP, ask for a printed list of doctors and clinics that can accommodate you in a day or two. If you do not have medical insurance, ask to speak with the social worker or head nurse. Many patients do end up returning to the ER for follow up care because of simple but avoidable oversights like the listed doctor does not accept your specific insurance plan. It is safest to fax over a copy of your insurance card to the doctor's office for approval.

- **Referral to a specialist who does not accept your insurance.** If your ailment requires specialist care, you might be referred directly to a specialist who was on-call for the emergency room that day. You are given a number to call for follow up care, but the specialist may not participate with your insurance plan. Now you must scramble to find a quality doctor for your needs who is on your health plan.

Solution: Solutions to find a specialist near your home may be difficult. Federal EMTALA laws require hospitals only to "stabilize" the emergency medical condition, but say nothing about who is responsible for final medical treatment. Possible situations: 1) Pay cash to specialist. Get the name of the on-call specialist, and have the ER physician contact the doctor to discuss your illness and give them your name. You can tell the receptionist the next day the two doctors agreed that you must be seen. 2) Get good insurance that most physicians accept. 3) Call your insurance plan and try to get an exception to use that specialist as "in-network" and therefore covered since the emergency room referred you. Ask to speak with a supervisor if you cannot get a reasonable override but this approach will not be easy to accomplish.

- **Beware prescriptions sent electronically to the wrong pharmacy:** Many ERs now send prescriptions electronically. They may be sent to a pharmacy miles across town or to one that is already closed.

Solution: If the hospital has an open pharmacy, have the prescription electronically sent there. Otherwise, use the closest 24-hour pharmacy for all your needs. You might prefer asking for a legible, *written* prescription so you can drop it off at any pharmacy. Before you walk out the door, check for accuracy of medication(s), dose, readability, length of supply, proper patient name, doctor signature and DEA number for controlled substances.

- **Not sending your PCP a copy of the ER visit:** You have a follow up appointment a few days after an ER visit with your primary care physician. In order for the PCP to best manage your care they will need to know what was done during the emergency visit. Any laboratory tests, imaging results, treatments rendered, and medications prescribed? Getting a hold of those records will then be delayed, and possibly overlooked.

Solution: Ask the ER physician to fax to your PCP a copy of key test results done in the emergency room. This might be a good bridge until the medical records department is able to send a complete ER visit record a couple weeks later.

- Getting **false reassurance** when rushed out of a busy emergency room. For example, a middle-aged woman suffering from bad indigestion goes to an ER because she is worried about a stomach ulcer. An ultrasound is ordered to exclude gallstones. She is then prescribed acid-lowering medication. "Tests are all okay so you are good to go," she is told. In truth, she had little relief with acid-lowering medication and continues to feel pain as she heads out those large metal ER doors. This woman, in fact, was a victim of false reassurance. She was subjected to a rushed evaluation with the main goal of emptying out the emergency department. The doctor spent more time ordering tests than speaking to and examining the lady. ER chaos and doctor exhaustion contributed to him heading down the wrong diagnostic path. He pursued abdominal illness and never considered her abdominal symptoms were actually caused by heart disease. *Key lesson*: never assume all is okay if told tests are normal but you continue to feel miserable. If ER treatments offer no benefit, perhaps doctors are barking up the wrong tree. *The* **solution:** have the physician in charge evaluate you as well. If necessary, insist you do not feel well enough to go home and perhaps need a specialist's expert opinion. Ask for the hospital's patient representative to come assist you if needed.

- **Lacking needed home health or hospice services** to properly assist and monitor you. Once again, do not allow discharge until all needed follow up care and services are properly in place. Be sure the home health agency participates with your insurance plan and can visit you quickly after your return home. If needed, have a doctor appointment set up already, preferably a home visit. Clarify if you require any infusion services or physical therapy for continued skilled care at home. Be sure all intravenous medication orders are clearly relayed to your follow up doctor.

INDEX

D

E

F

G

H

I

L

M

N

O

P

Q

R

S

BULK PURCHASE DISCOUNTS AVAILABLE

BoomER Emergency Room Survival Guide offers a treasure trove of basic care principles for older adults and frail elders. The book can serve as an educational tool for students in healthcare fields, paid and family caregivers, and those who care for older adults in nursing homes, assisted living and home-based settings. Hospices and home health agencies should use BoomER as continuing education credit for their professional and allied healthcare staff.

BoomER makes a useful and valuable gift of membership for geriatric, caregiver and healthcare organizations as well.

Libraries can purchase this book for all branches to fill a void in the niche of useful health advice for Baby Boomers and those caring for the growing elderly demographic.

Go to www.endlessknotpress.com or

www.emergencyroomsurvivalbookforolderadults.com for information on bulk purchases.

Any questions? Call 480-818-7845 or email us at endlessknotpress@gmail.com.

ABOUT THE AUTHORS

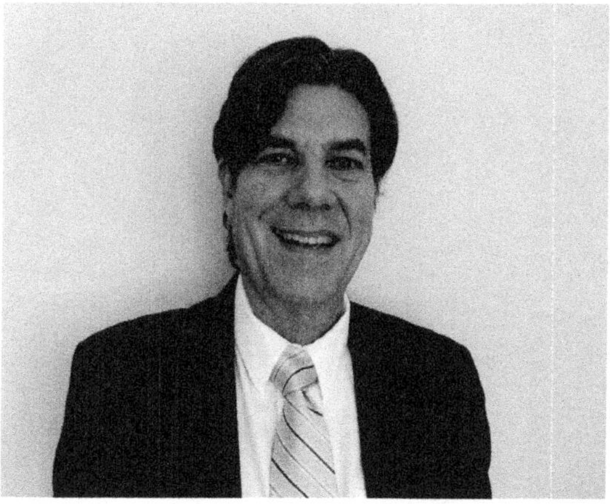

Robert W. Derlet, MD

Dr. Derlet is Professor Emeritus at the University of California, Davis School of Medicine, and former Chief of Emergency Medicine at the Davis Medical Center for nearly two decades. Dr. Derlet was also instrumental in starting the residency training program in emergency medicine. He has published over 100 scientific research articles on such topics as emergency room overcrowding and wilderness medicine. Dr. Derlet has lectured extensively both nationally and internationally, serving as visiting professor at numerous hospitals worldwide. He has provided care to patients on six out of seven continents.

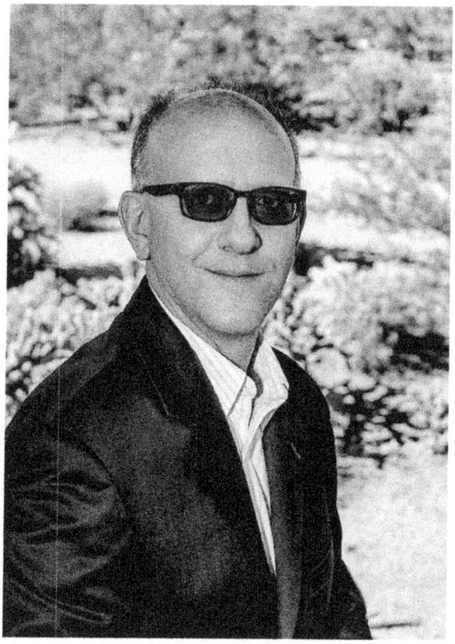

Joel Cohen, MD

Dr. Cohen serves as Medical Director of a highly regarded geriatric house call practice for needy seniors based in Scottsdale, Arizona. He has also previously practiced emergency and urgent care medicine for 10 years. Dr. Cohen has used his extensive experience and expertise to train nurse practitioners and teach medical, naturopathic and nurse practitioner students for over a decade. He is also Publisher and Senior Medical Editor of Endless Knot Press, LLC, a unique publishing company focused on solutions for health concerns of Baby Boomers and older adults. Dr. Cohen envisions a day when caring for older folks emphasizes quality of life, activity engagement, compassion, and hand-holding above medication-worship and test and procedure overuse.

Made in the USA
Monee, IL
04 November 2026

67385382R00187